NEUROLOGY ROUNDS WITH THE MAVERICK:

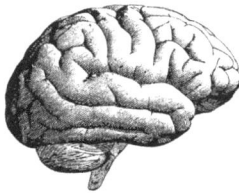

Adventure with Patients
from the Golden Age
of Medicine

By Bernard M. Patten, MD

IDENTITY PUBLICATIONS

Bernard M. Patten

———

AB (Columbia College summa cum laude)
MD (College of Physicians and Surgeons, Columbia University)
Fellow of the American College of Physicians
Fellow of the Royal Society of Medicine
Fellow of the Texas Neurological Society
Fellow of the American Academy of Neurology
Certified by the American Board of Psychiatry and Neurology

Copyright © 2019 Bernard M. Patten

All rights reserved. No part of this publication may be reproduced, distributed, or transmitted in any form or by any means, including photocopying, recording, or other electronic or mechanical methods, without the prior written permission of the publisher, except in the case of brief quotations embodied in critical reviews and certain other noncommercial uses permitted by copyright law. Any perceived slight against any individual is purely unintentional.

For permission requests, write to the publisher at:
contact@identitypublications.com

Ordering Information:

Quantity sales. Special discounts are available on quantity purchases by corporations, associations, and others. For details, contact the publisher at the address above.

Orders by U.S. trade bookstores and wholesalers. Please contact Identity Publications: Tel: (805) 259-3724 or visit www.IdentityPublications.com

ISBN-13: 978-1-722231-43-9 (paperback)
ISBN-13: 978-1-945884-64-1 (hardcover)

First Edition
Publishing by Identity Publications
www.IdentityPublications.com

Photos and documents referenced in this book are available on Dr. Patten's YouTube channel: www.YouTube.com/User/SuperMickey8888

"The old doctor who used to cure all sorts of diseases has completely disappeared. I assure you, now there are only specialists. ….If anything is wrong with your nose, they send you to Paris; there, they say, is a European specialist who cures noses. If you go to Paris, he'll look at your nose. I can only cure your right nostril, he'll tell you, for I don't cure the left nostril, that's not my specialty, but go to Vienna, there there's a specialist who will cure your left nostril."
Dostoyevsky

"All intellectual work builds on the ideas of others and influences those who follow."
John Carey
Fordham University

"People do not watch Bonanza to find out about the Old West."
Tony Schwartz
The Responsive Chord, 1973

Table of Contents

General Conversation
with the Reader

———

Some years ago—never mind how many—I gave a silver dollar to Shae Mia Patten, my granddaughter, who ran wide-eyed and skipping to her daddy and asked, "What is this?" He told her, "That is a coin of a bygone era."

For some time, Craig's statement bothered my sleep. But now I know it is true and not only that—I know I am from a bygone era, an era when life was quite different, an era that included what is now considered by doctors as the golden age of medicine. It was an interesting time for doctors because there were few administrators, the insurance companies did not interfere with medical practice, and, believe it or not, money was not a big issue. There was less technology so doctors relied on, had to rely on, taking a history and doing a physical examination, both of which gave close contact with their fellow human beings who were patients.

In the golden age, physicians became involved in the stories of their patients' lives, sometimes as witnesses and most times as players. It was a time when doctors knew their fellow creatures better than most men, knew the inner life which so seldom unfolds itself to unanointed eyes and ears. It was a time when medicine was a calling, not a job.

My own life, by being close to patients, by knowing their psychology deeply, has been entwined with patient lives and their stories. Thus, this is not my memoir alone but a memoir of the people I have known. One of the great benefits to a medical career is you get an endless fund of stories, some funny, some terrible— but all real.

The narrated events displayed in this book are true. They are a selected part of my curriculum vitae. They are not *based on* true events. They *are* the true events. If you are looking for fiction, you are reading the wrong book. Go watch TV.

Though this book is part of the literature of fact (there are no composite or made-up characters, nothing that isn't real or didn't happen), the names of some patients, as a courtesy, have been changed. But in the record about the breast implants, where there were problems aplenty, all the names are those of real people and all the events happened, including the raid on my laboratory, the death threats, the assault of Trent, my chauffeur, the beheaded rabbit at the doorstep, and the arson that burned down my nurse's home.

Part of even the most normal of us passes, during our lives, into a weird haunted chamber. My haunted chamber was the medical research on breast implants. In that haunted chamber, I became the classic historian, because I was there, and I lived through the horrors and the mess. The ladies who suffered from breast implants deserve to have their stories generally known, and that is exactly what I shall do in part three of this book.

So, if you continue to read, you will get a decentralized story, a narration of events in time, morally, and otherwise floating like a balloon over hullabaloo. Here you will see and I hope actually experience scenes of joy, sorrow, suffering, disease, ordeal and triumph, the real-life adventures of taking care of very sick people, the bummer of getting involved with malpractice lawsuits, as well as the battles entailed by standing up to corporate America in the matter of the safety and effectiveness of breast implants. As a physician, I took an oath to not only take care of the individual patient but to also protect the public health. Fighting powerful interests such as insurance companies and medical device manufacturers can mean being viewed as a weirdo, an outsider. That's the downside, but one that you have to be willing to accept.

About the Stories

————

There are a million ways to tell a story. You know there are. One way is chronological. Another way is by topic. Another way is by memory links as one story suggests or reminds of another. My way is to do all three and let it flow as normal people think most of the time and sometimes sprawl, telling you what's on their minds. And that's that. The approach is sensible and humane. So here I faithfully report to you, dear reader, scenes, events, and adventures in a privileged world that was in intimate contact with the nuance and foibles of human nature.

Enough!

In the final analysis, it is best to let the memoir speak for itself. That we shall do in the pages that follow.

But first a word of thanks to my wife.

Ethel—her title should be Saint Ethel—she truly loves me and has proved her love by living with me for the last 55 years. It is to her this work is dedicated. She doesn't need to read this book. She lived it. TO ETHEL: SINE TE NIHIL.

ATTENTION:
Why You Should Read This Book

———

Knowledge of the coming facts and events should bring you a sense and perception of a life and a world you might not have been otherwise familiar with. You may even be motivated to help make things improve. So, step up. Increase the intensity and range of your experience. Use this memoir as a source of knowledge to examine and clarify your life, the lives of others, and life in general. In the end, decide for yourself if it is better for a doctor to function at the junction of art and science and practice medicine NOT AS A STRANGER, or is it better for a doctor to enter the survival mode, knuckle under, and muddle through as many burned-out physicians are doing right now, as your own doctor, much to your detriment, might be doing right now. Decide: is it better to let your insurance company make medical decisions for you or better to let your doctor?

"When Dr. James D. Watson spoke at the Research Corporation dinner where he was honored for his work on DNA, many in the audience were startled by the account he gave of his career as a scientist. They expected a story of gradual discovery by orderly experiments and unfolding truths. They were prepared for setbacks of a technical kind which would retard but also heighten the final triumph. They were not prepared for the red thread of life which Watson wove into his narrative—the chance meetings and clashing personalities, the haste and envy, the fumbling and idling, in a word the politics and social vicissitudes of science."

Jacques Barzum
Science: The Glorious Entertainment

Record One:
Adventures and Misadventures in the Golden Age of Medicine

So, one day in 1988, I was making rounds with the students and residents, and a student presented me "the brain tumor in 209." And I said: "Isn't there a child involved in this? Tell me about the child. Tell me about the family. Do you know any of this?" They did not.

At home that night, Arnold Gold told his wife of his concerns about where medicine was headed. She told him, "You know, Arnold, I'm tired of you griping about medicine. Do something about it or shut up."

Thus, Arnold Gold, pediatric neurologist, made compassionate care a cause and founded the Arnold P. Gold Foundation to inspire young doctors to practice compassionate patient care. On rounds, he wanted doctors to know about the lives of their patients, not just their vital signs, not just the details of the disease afflicting them. *

*Abstracted from the New York Times obituary by Richard Sandomir, February 4, 2018.

Index to Patient Experiences

College of Physicians and Surgeons, Columbia University—1962-1966, New York City
Cornell Medical School, New York Hospital, 1966-1967
Neurological Institute of New York, 1967-1970
Moonlighting at University Heights Hospital, Bronx, New York City—1968,
National Institutes of Health 1970-1973, Bethesda, Maryland
Baylor College of Medicine, 1973-1996, Houston, Texas

Ready? Set!
Let's make rounds.

Tableau One:

The Kid Who Couldn't Stop Laughing and the Artist Who Was Losing His Mind

Patient Linda—Baylor College of Medicine
Uncontrollable Laughing

She was 15 and in high school. Her G.P. sent her because she was jerked out of French class because she couldn't or wouldn't stop laughing. "Was this a seizure disorder or a form of epilepsy?" the family physician asked.

The laughing started in the schoolyard in back of the handball court about halfway into the after-lunch recess. The laughing continued into French class and down at the principal's office. The uncontrolled and uncontrollable laughing stopped at 3:17 p.m. that afternoon. There have been no further episodes.

Linda's neurological examination was normal. To the concerned parents, I said, "I would like to talk with Linda alone. Please excuse us."

Attention reader: your diagnosis, please. How would you handle this situation and this patient? How would you handle her family?

Still with me? I pause for reply to make sure you are awake and to give you a chance to stretch your mental powers. What caused the uncontrolled laughing? What should be done?

Me: "Linda, I am going to let you off this time because I'm a nice guy. But promise me you won't smoke weed before school or at recess. That way you won't embarrass yourself again."

Linda: "I had never smoked that stuff before, but I didn't want to look like a chicken, so when the blunt came my way I took a long deep drag like a regular cigarette. I passed it to Lynette when the weed kicked in, and I couldn't stop laughing. I was laughing so hard I nearly keeled over. Nothing was funny, but I couldn't stop."

Me: "OK. Keep your mouth shut while I explain to your parents there is nothing to worry about. You're off the hook—this time."

"Linda is normal neurologically. Actually, quite intelligent."

Linda's father: "How do you know?"

"Detailed neurological exam is normal, so I know her nervous system is normal. She has an excellent thought process, fluent speech, and an advanced vocabulary, so I know she is intelligent.

"The laughing episode will probably never happen again. She doesn't have a seizure disorder, and even if she did, we wouldn't treat her or anyone, for that matter, for a single seizure. If we treated people for a single isolated seizure, 3% of the population of America would be taking seizure medicines. So, no tests, no treatment. Go home and forget it."

The High School Syndrome

Linda's case is part of a larger syndrome of high school kids asleep in class or drunk. The usual cause is alcohol or drugs. The laughing problem is almost always due to marijuana smoked just before school starts or at recess. Strangely, the laughing fits seem to involve only teenage girls. As far as I know, the syndrome was never written up in the neurology journals. It's too trivial. Experienced neurologists would make the correct diagnosis without much thinking. No tests needed. The diagnosis is secure, as it often is, just from the history alone.

George Rodrigue—Artist and Painter
Subacute Dementia

A young artist came to see me because he was losing his mind. He had painted several paintings that had sold for a lot of money, and, though he was young, he already had a national and international reputation for his work. His most famous paintings involved an iconic painting of a blue dog, the shape and stance of which was based on his deceased dog, Tiffany, and on the Cajun legend of a loup-garou or werewolf.

The problem was over the course of a year George had noticed a fall-off in his creative abilities, and he had noticed his memory was failing. On more than a few occasions, he would start to say something and then forget what he was talking about. Despite a valiant effort, he just couldn't get back to the subject. Whole evenings would slip out of consciousness, never to be recalled again. This kind of memory deficit is much more serious than ordinary forgetting. It is one thing to forget what you ate for dinner and another quite different thing to forget you had dinner at all.

"George, I am going to say three items. Store them in your memory. I will ask you what they were in about three minutes. Here's the items: 979 San Lorenzo, National Football League, Jones Beach.

"George, how much is 3 plus 2?"

George looks at me as if I'm crazy for asking such a stupid question.

The Kid Who Couldn't Stop Laughing and the Artist Who Was Losing His Mind

"Five!"

"That's correct. Now tell me. what were the three items I asked you to remember?

George shakes his head. Not only does he not recall the items, he doesn't remember my asking him to remember.

"George, how much is 5 minus 3?"

George is truly puzzled. He can't say or guess. Nor can he do 7 minus 4, or 5 minus 4.

"George, spell *cat*."

"C-A-T."

"Good. Correct! Now spell *cat* backward."

George looks puzzled. He doesn't get the task even though I explain in detail cat spelled forward is C-A-T, and I want him to start with the last letter of cat and work backward to the second letter and then the first. Try as he must, he can't do it. Nor can he spell *world* backward or *park*. Nor can he tell me whether or not I have spelled those words backward.

"Why can't he spell backward? Why can't he do the stupid subtractions?" asks his wife.

"A fair question. The short answer is we don't know. The long answer is people with organic brain diseases can't spell simple words backward and they can't do simple subtractions. Difficulty in doing such tasks is characteristic of memory problems associated with brain damage, particularly damage to the temporal lobes of the brain."

And so, dear reader, if you can spell cat backward and subtract 3 from 5, I give it for my opinion as a board-certified neurologist you are not demented—not yet.

Except for impairment of ability to remember, poor ability to mentally subtract numbers, and inability to spell simple words like "cat" backward, his neurological examination was OK. Family history, social history, and personal history were OK, except he was drinking a quart of rye whiskey every night.

The brain scan (this was the era of CAT scan) showed tremendous loss of brain tissue with dilated ventricles (the fluid-filled cavities in the center of the brain), narrow gyri, and enlarged sulci (the gyri are brain tissue ridges and the sulci the valleys between ridges).

Dilated ventricles usually mean loss of brain tissue, narrow gyri (ditto), enlarged sulci (ditto). Result: the CAT scan showed severe decrease in brain size, presumably due to severe loss of brain tissue itself.

"Looking at the scan, George, I estimate you have lost over 40% of your brain. That's not good."

George looks at the scan and strokes his chin. He is examining the image in great detail but says nothing. What is he thinking? What?

"George, the prognosis is not good. In fact, it is grim. Get ready to lose your mind. Make arrangements for your care when you become demented. Prepare while you can. This is frightening, I know, but you have to get things ready and in order."

"Doc, what's causing the problem?"

"Who knows? Drinking a quart of rye whiskey a day, every day is probably not helping."

Yes, that is what he said he drank, and there is no reason to think he was bragging. If anything, at least according to his wife, he might have been underestimating the dose of booze. A quart of whiskey a day would be a big dose even by the standards of my Irish family. It is probably a big dose by Cajun standards as well.

"If you continue to drink like that," says I, "you will soon be dead."

Notice I did not say, "You must stop drinking." That kind of medical advice is paternalistic and takes part of the patient's personal power away. This man is an adult, and he has to decide what he wants to do with his life. My job, as I saw it at the time, was to give advice in the form of a realistic warning about death.

"Death is a bad thing, George," I told him. "It spoils your weekend."

And then to emphasize the seriousness of the situation, I showed and explained the CAT scan to him in detail. He was impressed by the visual image of his rotted brain, much more impressed by the picture than he was by my warning in words. After all, the man is an artist, a great artist. Pictures spoke to him louder than words. And his pictures spoke to other people louder than words. Then he asked what I thought was a rather naïve question.

"Will my brain grow back?"

"Certainly not! Brain tissue, once lost, is lost forever. The best you may hope for is to arrest the brain loss at the present level. Your brain will never recover, for it never can recover. That is a fact. The brain does not repair itself."

Why I Delivered Complete Hokum and Bullshit

At the time, that hokum is what neurologists believed to be true. My advice was right in line with the standard of care for that time and place. Anything less would have been considered wrong by my peers, by the Texas Board of Medical Examiners, and by the American Board of Psychiatry and Neurology. The dogma the brain can't recover was not in a gray zone. It was considered a fact, a piece of received standard wisdom, irrefutable gospel-level truth. In that era, erroneous ideas were passed, like religious writ, from one generation to another, from one medical article to another.

The dogma of the inability of the brain to recover is now passé—part of a bygone era, like myself and like the silver dollar I gave to Shae Mia Patten, my granddaughter. George was justified not to take my word. He was justified to demand proof his brain would not recover.

"How do you know for sure my brain can't recover?"

"George, every neurology textbook and every professor of neurology and almost all of the neurologists of the world say so. We must accept the opinion of the authorities."

My trouble was I was a victim of conjecture because during medical school, internship, and residency, my professors told me what they thought was fact. So, I continued to try to get this point across by making mere assertions I myself had never even thought to question. I was very dumb in those days. I still am dumb but not as much. Mark Twain famously said, "It is not what I don't know that hurts. It is all the things I think I know that ain't true." I was sure the brain did not repair itself as other human organs and human tissues do, but it so happens that ain't true. So, at the time, I continued to feed George bullshit I thought was the truth.

Me: "Once brain tissue is lost, it can never be recovered."

What I did in advising this patient was merely repeat poll-parrot style the neurological dogma drummed into my head during my medical training. At the time, it was considered no more possible to regenerate brain tissue than it was possible to fly to the moon. Now humans can do both. Also, I know now that reiteration of a mere assertion is not proof of anything. Blindsided by an authority argument I was. Now I ask for evidence. If the evidence is not relevant and adequate, I will not believe the assertion. It's that simple and an important lesson. Doubt and skepticism are important parts of thinking like a scientist.

In ancient times when dissections were done, they often showed the teachings of Galenic medicine were wrong. And yet, the evidence was dismissed as accidental or fake. The medical system thus rejected medical science and what Shakespeare called "ocular proof" as irrelevant. Even in the early days of my medical education, medicine, some of it anyway, was still a branch of theology, wherein you accepted doctrines on faith, a big mistake.

Yet another example: when I was an intern, the tradition dictated that patients who had heart attacks had to be placed on complete bed rest for four to six weeks to allow the injured heart to repair itself. Sitting in a chair was prohibited. Patients were not allowed to turn from side to side without assistance. The mortality with this treatment was about 35%, with a large number of victims dying from pulmonary embolism. In addition, about 67% of the patients developed frozen shoulders with swollen red left hands and arms, a condition that greatly impaired the patient's ability to dress. We were told the shoulder-hand syndrome was a reaction of the sympathetic nervous system to the heart attack. Some patients actually got their sympathetic nerves cut on that side without improvement. How did the professors explain the lack of improvement after sympathectomy? They said, "Well, it was just too late." Or they said, "We see it." Never was there any mention of the idea that failure to respond to the operation meant the premise of the operation was in error, and the shoulder-hand problem had nothing whatsoever to do with heart attacks or with the sympathetic nervous system.

Complete bed rest also meant no bathroom privileges. Each patient had to use the bedpan, and every time they went the nurses had to move the patient on and off the pan. Nurses also fed the patients three times a day. Think of the inconvenience of that and the embarrassment. Think of the amount of nursing work involved.

When some physicians proposed chair rest, not bed rest, for heart attack victims, the idea met with a dust storm of tremendous resistance from tradition-oriented doctors. Initial studies were not approved by institutional review committees.

Nevertheless, some pioneering physicians went ahead (this, remember, was the era wherein the individual doctor had total control of his/her individual patient). Those doctors dared to get their heart attack patients out of bed and into a chair. The results were obvious from the get-go. From the very first patient, chair rest made all the difference. Mortality declined to 10%. Frozen shoulder-hand syndrome disappeared completely because it was due to disuse and had nothing whatever to do with the sympathetic nervous system or even with the heart attack. Pulmonary embolism became a rare event. Pneumonia from immobilization even became far less frequent.

Now we know bed rest is harmful for a number of reasons: it rots bones and weakens muscles. But the worst thing about it, in my view, is the mental and psychological demoralization that comes with remaining in bed 24/7. After all, in America, most of the dying takes place in bed, and there is a sense of safety in being out of bed.

Although there has never been and never will be a double-blind prospective controlled study comparing bed rest with chair rest for heart attack, chair rest is now the standard of care, and bed rest is not.

The way doctors rationalized treatments without merit was draconian and still troubles my sleep. It is creepy to realize many medical practices are not soundly based, but instead are supported by inertia, fashion, custom, tradition, and undue respect for authority. Long-held belief systems, even when not backed by evidence, become proof of validity and a tremendous impediment to progress. At present, I point the finger of accusation at the oncologists who tend to intervene no matter what the human costs. Usually they are truthful about defining the small chance of success, but they have not been as forthright about the miserable consequences of chemotherapy. Better to manage the incurable with common sense and compassion. Sometimes the health care system is structured to torture the elderly, not because of malevolence but because it is a program based on reimbursement rather than what is best for the patient. My 95-year-old mother-in-law gave it for her opinion, "Sometimes doctors do what isn't needed because Medicare will pay."

How's that for insight!

> **Lesson:** Sometimes, the concepts we think we know so well, that have become part of us, and, automatically part of our consciousness, are wrong. We need to change them every so often, not just general, social, political, or philosophical concepts, but also, at times, scientific and medical concepts as well. Otherwise, there will be little or no progress.

What happened next?

Three months later, George, the artist returned for a follow-up examination. He felt he had recovered. His wife gave it for her opinion, "George is thinking better than ever."

My examination confirmed his thinking, memory, and even the subtractions were now not only normal but superior. He spelled long words backward without any trouble. What had happened? Why and how did George recover?

The Answer

He stopped the booze.

Remove the cause of a disease, and you usually get an improvement, and his improvement was dramatic. Fantastic really!

"Doc, I'm back to my old self. But what happened to my brain? Can we do another scan?"

"Sorry, George. A repeat scan would be a waste of time and money. It will show no change because the brain can't grow back."

"How do we know for sure?"

"George, it is so sure the brain can't grow back that I am sure your insurance company will not pay for a repeat scan. Why should they when it is a known fact the brain cannot regenerate?"

Sure enough, as predicted, the insurance company wouldn't pay for another scan, but the patient himself did pay the $850 (scans were cheaper in those days, and money was more valuable).

George wanted to see the picture of his brain again, and he was willing to pay to foot the bill, an attitude consistent with his vocation as a visual artist who felt seeing is believing. Here was a patient who had to know. He had to see it to believe it. And the money meant very little to him, as he was already a multimillionaire thanks to the Blue Dog paintings.

A person's profession can affect how he or she sees things. An architect or a plumber may see the structure and pipes of a building, whereas an artist would be attracted by the building's form. Nazzi, the woman who cuts my hair, knows much more about my hair than I do. She takes a professional interest in hair and in my hair that I don't. When I see people limping on the street, I can usually tell exactly what is wrong and why they are limping because appraising gait is a detailed part of the training of all neurologists.

Result

George was right: seeing is believing. If you see something, you believe it. If you don't see it, you don't know. Seeing is believing. But if you don't see it, does that mean it isn't there, and you shouldn't believe it?

Aye, there's the rub. It could be there, and you missed it. Or the tools you are using could have been wrong for that particular observation. For instance, if I say there are no bacteria on this paper, and I am using a telescope to look for the bacteria, I will be using the wrong tool and reaching the wrong conclusion. You can't see bacteria with a telescope. To see bacteria, you need a microscope, not a telescope. There are billions of bacteria on this book and on your pillow at night. You can't see them. But they are there. The general rule is seeing is believing, and the absence of evidence is not evidence of absence. In other words, if you don't see something, you just don't know. If you just don't know, it is better to suspend judgment until more evidence appears and justifies a conclusion. That way, you will not make the error of believing something not true. Think like a scientist. Demand evidence. Don't over exercise the believing parts of your brain.

The Artist's CAT Scan Result:
the Brain Scan is Normal, as Normal as the Patient!

George's brain, which had been three sizes too small, was now normal in size and shape and internal structure. Why it was normal and why it recovered is another question. He stopped the booze. My opinion is that dose of alcohol each day disturbed protein metabolism in his brain and made the brain appear small. But all of the adverse effects of the alcohol must have been reversible because they did reverse when he stopped drinking. Another possibility was the alcohol had dehydrated the brain, making it appear small because the water content had been reduced. The brain is over 90% water, so a decrease in water content would make the brain appear small. Isn't it remarkable the human brain, an organ that is mostly water, can do any kind of thinking!

An Earthquake

The ground shook. The foundation of neurological training at the great Neurological Institute of New York collapsed in a pile of dust with this personal earthquake. In logic, to disprove a general statement wrong all that is needed is one true counter-example. For instance, if I say all swans are white, and you show me a black swan (as exist in Russia) then the statement is proven wrong. The statement that the brain never regenerates is proven wrong by the one contrary example, demonstrated by George's demand for a repeat scan. More power to him. He taught me a lesson, a great lesson, a lesson that gave me the feeling artists, under some circumstances, can and do teach doctors a great deal.

> **Lesson:** The brain, like so many other body organs, just like so many other body tissues, has the potential to recover. Under the right circumstances, it will recover. And in this case, it did recover. It recovered functionally as evidenced by the artist's mental status examination, and the brain recovered structurally as evidenced by the repeat CAT scan that was now normal.

> **Lesson:** Much of medicine in the old days was unproven conjecture handed down from professors to students, with no real scientific evidence to back up the conjecture. Instead of science, neurology was a kind of religion based on faith. Whether medicine is still unscientific or not, I don't know. I have a feeling progress has been made, but not that much.

> **Lesson:** Absence of evidence is not evidence of absence. If you see it, you may believe it. If you don't see it, you don't know. If you don't know, then suspend judgment.

Since then, scans have proved the point time and time again, so we are sure of the fact diseased nervous tissue, given the right circumstances, can recover, re-grow, and look normal and be normal. We know that fact for sure because we can see it displayed on the scans.

Yep, such is the answer for diseased brain tissue. It also raises serious questions about the diagnosis of so-called brain death. To declare a brain is dead because it appears dead, begs the question and merely asserts what needs to be proven.

When I was an intern at the New York Hospital, I took care of a young woman who had a flat line electroencephalogram (EEG). She had taken a massive overdose of a long-acting barbiturate, Seconal, and then changed her mind and called for help. Help arrived just as she slipped into coma, and artificial respiration was started immediately.

Seconal is also known as secobarbital. The street name is "red devils" or "reds" because of the orange/red 100 mg bullet-shaped capsule. The other nickname was "dolls" which was partly responsible for the title of Jacqueline Susann's novel *Valley of the Dolls*, wherein the major character uses and abuses this drug as many people did in the 1960s to 1970s. Recall, at age 36, Marilyn Monroe, after a life of depression and failed marriages, died of a Seconal overdose in 1962. Actress Carole Landis checked out in the same way probably for the same reasons.

Karen's Overdose and Failed Suicide

On admission to the New York Hospital Karen's electroencephalogram was a flat line. No electrical activity was detected in her brain, and therefore, many of my fellow physicians thought Karen was brain dead. I thought the only thing the flat line EEG proved was there was no detectable brain electrical activity. It didn't prove her brain was dead, because the drug was obviously suppressing nervous system activity—it was producing coma. Why couldn't a massive blood level of barbiturate also suppress the EEG? So despite the claims I was wasting medical resources, I kept Karen alive by managing electrolytes, controlling infections, feeding her with IVs and a nasogastric tube, and, most importantly, keeping her on the respirator.

The human brain requires minute-to-minute supplies of oxygen. If the respirator were turned off, Karen's brain would have died six minutes later, and the autopsy would have confirmed brain death. In that case, the autopsy would have appeared to confirm the idea that the flat EEG did, in fact, indicate the brain was dead.

Get it? If you don't understand this, reread the paragraph. Pay particular attention to the idea of begging the question. We should not assume something is true (like brain death) unless proven. That the brain *appears* dead is not proof it is dead. It may just look dead. The EEG, in this case, was the wrong tool to appraise brain death.

> **Lesson:** This is important: turning off the respirator makes the brain dead. It doesn't prove the brain was dead before the respirator was turned off.

The nurses did a wonderful job turning Karen, cleaning up after incontinence, protecting from bed sores, etc. Without nurses and without my care, Karen would not have had a chance to survive.

Over the next six weeks, the blood level of barbiturate gradually declined because the liver was metabolizing the drug. Karen awoke and was normal. Yes, normal. Even her EEG was normal. Her grateful father made a donation to the medical center, and Karen and her family thought I was a hero.

"I'm no hero, Karen. I was just doing my job. You caused me and the nurses lots of extra bloody work. Next time you try to kill yourself, do it right."

How About Normal Brain Tissue?

But what about normal brain tissue? Can we, by directed mental activity, grow brain tissue to suit a particular need? The answer is yes, yes, yes! Playing the piano for two weeks will expand the areas of the brain involved. The London Taxi Cab study showed people studying to be taxi drivers in London increase the size of the brain structure (right parietal lobe) involved in navigation on London roads.

Follow-Up of Our Artist Patient

George Rodrigue's subsequent career speaks for itself. He went on to produce many famous paintings, and he donated much to charities.

In June 2008, the New Orleans Museum of Art had a George Rodrigue retrospective that broke the museum's attendance record for an exhibition of work by a living artist. More than 6,000 visitors flocked to the museum during the exhibit's closing weekend on June 7-8, bringing total attendance to 52,813 during the exhibit's 14-week run.

Sad to say, this very good artist, and very good man, died in Houston during the winter of 2013 at age 69. The lung cancer that killed him was caused, in his view, by the chemical sprays he used in his work.

It is certain George Rodrigue will get into heaven.

All he has to do is offer a Blue Dog painting to God.

Tableau Two:
The Old Lady Who Needed a Hug

Baylor College of Medicine
Patient Gertrude

Her name was Gertrude, and she lived in Port Arthur, Texas. She had a problem with a rare disease called Myasthenia Gravis. When I first saw her in clinic, she was having double vision, trouble talking, chewing and swallowing, and was feeling weak. Her condition was much better in the mornings when she first got up and got worse as the day wore on. Exercise made her worse, and rest made her better. Examination showed the usual for myasthenia: droopy eyelids, muffled low-pitched voice, easy fatigue of muscles, and so forth. Her condition responded to the usual treatments, and she regained her health and returned to normal on minimal amounts of prednisone, the standard treatment for her type of myasthenia. Eventually, the dose of prednisone was reduced to three milligrams on alternate days, and she remained in remission as long as she took that dose. If the dose was reduced to two milligrams on alternate days, she had trouble chewing and swallowing, and the fatigue returned.

She felt she had been saved from death and wanted to make sure the disease stayed under control. So every year she returned to clinic for a check-up, and after each clinic visit, she would stand up and ask to be hugged. I always hugged her. After all, she was over 80 years old and could have been my grandmother, and, more importantly, she needed a hug.

This scenario continued for years until a lecturer from the Texas Medical Board came to talk to us about medical ethics. The board requires every licensed physician in Texas to complete continuing medical education, and part of the requirement involves education about ethics. The lecturer gave it, for his opinion, there should be no personal contact at any time, for any reason between a physician and the patient. Hugging a patient was strictly unethical and forbidden.

Whew! That was news. How strange was it for me to listen to a young man with a background in business administration tell me not to socialize with my patients. When the lecture was over, it was time for questions, and I had one.

"For the last 30 years, my dentist would repair my teeth in the morning and then take me to his country club and treat me to lunch. Was that wrong? At lunch, he and I discussed a long laundry list of our personal and family problems. Is that wrong? On my last visit, my dentist gave me an electric toothbrush. Was that wrong?"

"Report his unethical and very bad behavior to the Dental Board. Socializing with a patient is highly unethical as is giving gifts. Having lunch with a patient is a definite no-no!"

Whoa!

Of course, I had no intention to report my dentist friend. The Irish don't rat. You can rely on that. But there is an important issue here about trying to prevent exploitation of patients. The power relations between patient and doctor are sometimes out of balance, and some physicians have used their position to abuse patients. That was not the situation with my dentist friend. Nor do I think it was the situation with Gertrude.

Per usual, Gertrude returned to clinic for a check-up. She was fine. But at the end of her visit when she stood for her hug, she was told about the ethics lecture, the medical board, and the new constraints on me, her physician, about hugs.

"What no hug?" Gertrude asked.

I nodded yes—no hug. "I can't. It's against the law or something."

At this point mild-mannered Gertrude, my old grandmother-type patient, lost her cool and started shouting. "For God's sake, the only reason I come to clinic is for my hug. I'm not leaving until I get my hug. I need a hug. This is ridiculous."

Nurses ran into the examining room to find out what the commotion was about. Was Doctor Patten raping an old woman? Gertrude defiantly refuses to leave and her screaming is upsetting the 50-odd patients in the waiting room. Chaos and commotion. Real-life chaos and commotion, not something engineered by some hack writer of TV melodrama. Shall I make sense, or shall I tell the truth? Choose either. You can't have both. I shall not indulge in that primitive storytelling instinct, itself a hangover from religion, to retrospectively impose meaning on real-life chaos. No! No! No!

The truth is Gertrude is going ape shit over a trivial nothing. She is shouting hysterically simply because she is not getting her usual hug, a hug now forbidden by the exalted Texas Board of Medical Examiners. It is not her fault, and it is not my fault. But there is a problem. Gertrude will not leave the examining room. She won't leave clinic, and she will not stop shouting unless she gets a hug. That's it. Should I call security to remove her? Or should I violate the received standard of medical ethics and hug her?

To hug or not to hug? That is the question.

Reader, I ask you: what would you do?

The Old Lady Who Needed a Hug

Well, what would you do? What would you do? You, reader, I am asking you directly. What would you do?

I pause for reply.

And what do you think I should do?

I pause for reply.

And what do you think I did?

I hugged her of course. Both because she needed it, and I needed to get her out of clinic. After over four decades in medical practice, I have learned to give the patients what they (within reason) want.

Doctor and patient relationships are associated with a certain degree of intimacy. And, I suppose, there is a concern in making a firm distinction between the role of doctor and the role of lover. That is a crude concern. The condition under which Gertrude got her hug is sexually impossible. Her hug belongs to the experience of childhood. I hug her as I would hug my grandmother. With all she and I had been through together, all we had suffered together while she and I were desperately trying to get the myasthenia under control, I was an honorary member of her family. I had saved her life. Saving a life confers privileges. Does it not?

So I hugged her. So what! No harm done.

Gertrude got her hug and left clinic happy and satisfied, while I violated medical ethics and worried someone might rat.

It was a mistake for me to take the medical board's prescription as dogma. How could I be so stupid? Lewis Thomas, in *The Youngest Science*, comments, "touching is the oldest and most effective tool in doctoring." For me, this statement rings true. Too bad touching has become perfunctory as the physical examination has grown cursory. Medicine as a science has gone far. But scientific progress does not mandate ignoring those qualities that promote caring. Laying on the hands is necessary, lest medicine loses the close bond between doctor and patient.

Sidebar about My Image Consultant

Talking about touching patients reminded me of John T. Molloy, the image consultant I hired in 1973 to advise me about how to augment my medical practice. Molloy made rounds with me and watched me in clinic. He even stood in the visitors' gallery while I operated, and he interacted with patients and nurses and medical students. After three days of observation during which he took lots of notes, Molloy went into hiding for a week and came back with six single-spaced typed pages of advice.

John: "Cut your hair so you stop looking like a hippy." I was wearing hair hippy style down to my shoulder blades. I got a haircut, and the Houston police stopped stopping my car on the Gulf Freeway and no longer searched the car for drugs. The first month I was in Houston, I had been stopped four times. I had a license for any drug they would have found, but the cops didn't know that.

John: "Get rid of the thick glasses." I did and now wear contacts. I see better too.

John: "Never wear a bow tie. You look like a clown, and you need a regular tie as a contrast to the neurology department chairman."

John: "Don't loom over patients. When you enter a patient's hospital room, always greet her, touch her or shake hands, and sit down next to the bed or on the bed itself. This makes you look more human and neutralizes or tends to neutralize the high-tech atmosphere of the hospital. In general, patients are scared stiff and need and want tender loving care."

John: "Always touch the patient when you see them in clinic or in their room or in the operation (sic) room before you cut them up. Touch is human and reassures people, makes them feel safe, and lets them know you care. It is not enough they know they are safe; they have to feel safe, get on the emotional plane, and get off the intellectual plane. You and your practice are too scientific and too intellectual and not humane enough."

Of course, there was lots of other advice which need not concern us here. I paid John $600 and did what he recommended. Within six weeks, my practice quadrupled. Two years later, in 1975, P.H. Wyden published John's bestselling book, "Dress for Success." I love old books like this one for their occasional anachronisms and because the old authors generally are more sensible and much more honest. Take a look at the book and admire John's candor.

Back to Patient Gertrude

With Gertrude, the situation with repeated ethical violations on each and every clinic visit continued for three years. Then Gertrude had a stroke. Three days after her stroke, she died in Saint Elsewhere Hospital in Port Arthur while I was living it up on vacation in Italy at the Grand Hotel in Taormina, sipping an ice-cold Tanqueray martini while overlooking the eternal Ionian Sea that "sang in its chains," to quote Dylan Thomas. Swells and waves swaying to a not-quite-anapestic beat.

Good News and Bad News

Gertrude's death was bad news. But her lawyer had good news. Gertrude left her estate to me. Her will said Doctor Patten doesn't know anything about this, but she is leaving everything to me as proof she loves me. The evidence that constituted the proof consisted of her bank account with $105,000, her mortgage-free home, her Steinway D concert grand piano, multiple computers (Gertrude did software reviews for a hobby and for pay), and her personal diary. All assets came to me tax-free as an inheritance, proving hugging a patient can't be all bad.

Taking care of Gertrude was my job. But no patient ever thanked me more. But trouble was headed my way, and stupid me didn't even realize how bad that trouble would be.

Gertrude's Relatives Sue Doctor Patten

Gertrude's family contested the will. Not the money, not the house, not the Steinway D concert piano, not the computers, and so forth. The family wanted the diary and only the diary. Their lawyer explained it to me in my office. He had already filed the lawsuit, and he wanted me to know the family was dead set (pardon the expression—his words not mine) "They are dead set about the case. They want her diary."

In the evening after dinner, I read the first few pages. Although Gertrude might have been an old bag when she first came to clinic, she had a history. She played the piano for a night club and had extracurricular activities connected to the men she met there. Such stuff was not suitable for her relatives to know. If Gertrude would have wanted them to have the diary, she would have willed it to them and not to me. Gertrude left her diary for me to read because (I think) she wanted me to know she had had her fun and her moments of pleasure when she was young and in her salad days and green in judgment. She wanted me to know there was a time in her life and in the lives of others during which she raised hell. And she was proud of it. Way to go, Gertrude. Way to go!

After reading ten pages, I started to cry. Gertrude had lived a life well worth living. In clinic, she looked like an old bag, talked like an old bag, and walked like an old bag, because time and fate had kicked her in the face and laid her low, as I expect time will do to me. But the gentlemen she had loved were in her memory. In her diary, she had spit into the face of time that had transfigured her. In clinic, I would have never imagined Gertrude had such a history. But she did!

Turn Over the Diary or Don't Turn Over the Diary?
That is the Question...

What would you do, dear reader? Would you return the diary? I asked the question of six people. Each said without hesitation they would hand it over to the family. When I asked why, they said, "To get out of the lawsuit." When I asked those six people what they thought I did, each said they thought I turned the diary over to the family. When I asked why, they said, "To get out of the lawsuit."

Ignobly faint-hearted, pusillanimous nothings! No guts, no glory. O Tempora! O Mores! Sweet Jesus, I couldn't believe these people were such yellow-bellied cowards. They were afraid of a lawsuit. My creative writing instructor at Rice University even said, "I would rather have cancer, than a lawsuit." He got his wish. Soon thereafter, he contracted and died of acute leukemia. Never talk like that. It tempts the gods.

What I Did with the Diary

"Discretion is the better part of valor," to quote Falstaff. So I took the better part. I took the diary to the edge of my backyard and burned it. Burned the diary, that is, not the backyard.

The family was out of luck. They were never going to get the diary because the diary no longer existed. Even if they won the lawsuit, they couldn't recover the diary. There are distinct limits to the justice system. In most lawsuits, almost anything can happen, including nothing, as was the case here.

Result: the lawyer withdrew. And that was that.

Lesson: Hug them.

Lesson: No guts, no glory.

As stated, Gertrude had her stroke while I was on vacation in Italy. That reminds me of the experiences Ethel and I had during vacation.

Two Italian Men

Once two items are associated in the consciousness, each tends to recall the other and in the order first presented. Here the mention of Gertrude's stroke while I was at the hotel in Taormina triggered a memory of Italy and two Italian men. So the problem with this narrative is now, whether I should try to keep to some kind of order, chronological or logical, topical, or whatnot, or like Proust, just follow the patterns of my thoughts and tell, and not tell, as my spirit sees fit. There are a million ways of telling a story. You know there are. Others have their ways, and I have mine. The reason I write like this is this is the kind of thing I like to read. Not having seen this kind of stuff elsewhere, I create it for my own enjoyment, and I hope for your enjoyment and the enjoyment of others.

At Leisure in Italy

Taormina is a small town on the east coast of the island of Sicily, Italy. It is in the province of Messina, about midway between Catania and Messina, on the Ionian Sea, which, by the way, is warm with nice beaches. The majestic Grand Hotel Taormina stands on a cliff overlooking the hotel's private beach, and there were a nice garden and pool by the edge of the cliff and an aerial tramway that led down to the water. Whether the Grand Hotel Taormina still exists or not, and if it does exist whether it still has a tramway and private beach, I don't know, and I don't care, and I am too lazy to look it up. The Hotel's present existence is not relevant. This story is about a past adventure that happened there.

At the time of the appearance of Italian man one, the hotel and Taormina were very popular tourist attractions. That is why Ethel and I were there.

A Strange Interlude

One night, just as I sat down to dinner in the main dining room, the head waiter came to our table and asked if he could speak with me.

"Yes, of course."

"I want to fight you for your wife. I am in love with her."

I was sympathetic. Ethel is very lovable, and men do fall in love with her 'though not a word is spoken.

Me: "Fight? OK. But may I finish my dinner?"

He: "Of course. Meet me at 9:30 tonight in the garden by the pool, and we will fight."

"OK. 9:30 in the garden."

Ethel was amused by this. So was I. Ethel was always beautiful and sexy, so I could understand this guy's attitude (see photo). But surely, he was joking, and we continued dinner thinking his was a highly amusing joke.

Our amusement turned to chagrin when we arrived at the garden and saw the head waiter waiting. He was serious, and as he removed his jacket, he told me to get ready.

"OK." I looked him straight in the eyes and pointed my finger at his chest. "Before we start, I need to tell you in the United States I am considered a trained prizefighter. My trainer was my Uncle Tom, who was the middleweight champion of Queens, New York. If we fight, it is possible I will kill you."

Now the chagrin was his. He paused, developed a long face, a kiss-pout like a child rejecting the breast, wrinkled his brow, and announced with a shrug, "You can have her."

He left.

And that was that.

Lesson: The best battles are the ones you win without going toe to toe.

Italian Man Two

Two weeks later, we were in Ischia, a volcanic island in the Tyrrhenian Sea. It lies at the northern end of the Gulf of Naples and is situated northwest of Capri, which is better known, but not as nice. The main industry in Ischia is tourism centered around the thermal spas. And that is why Ethel and I were there.

In the mornings, Ethel and I would take breakfast on the veranda overlooking the pool and gardens of the Grand Hotel Ischia. From the first breakfast on, we became aware of a young man, Italian man two (Italian man one was the head waiter), staring at us. He stood leaning on a tree about 20 feet from the veranda and stayed there looking at us until our breakfast was over. He was an Adonis with curly blond hair and a fit body. When we left our table, he left his position and went I know not where.

In the afternoons, he was at the entrance to the hotel and followed us wherever we went. In the evenings, there was a carnival in town, and Ethel and I would walk to town to enjoy the sights and sounds of carnival. He followed us into town. He followed us around the carnival, he watched me win and lose at the games, and he followed us back to the hotel. In more modern times, he would have been considered a stalker. Come to think on it, he was a stalker, but in those days society didn't have a word for his behavior. We just thought he was a follower, and we couldn't think of a reason to stop him, and we couldn't think of a way to stop him.

Our young follower stalked us for three more days and nights. On day four, Ethel went inside the hotel to answer a telephone call. I stayed at poolside reading a book about the history of sex, a very interesting book about the history of sex in different cultures at different times. The varieties of sexual expression throughout history are enormous. It is a very good book. I recommend it for those few of you who might be interested in sex (title: *Sex in History* by Reay Tannahill, Stein and Day). Also by the same author: *Food in History*; and another book: *Flesh and Blood: A History of the Cannibal Complex.*

Back to poolside, as a deep, dark, shadow passes over the history of sex. I look up. The stalker is there looming over me, blocking the sunlight and interfering with my reading, just when I was getting into Tantric.

He smiles and speaks: "I suppose you noticed I have been following you. Do you understand my English?"

"Pretty good English. You do have a slight Italian accent, but I understand you and, yes, we have noticed you have been following us."

"And I suppose you know what I want?"

"Yes, I do. You want to fight me for my wife."

"No! I'm in love with you!"

I thanked him and explained I wasn't that kind of man. He got the long face, bowed out, and left. We didn't see him again. Ethel was amused and thought it was about time someone in Italy, besides herself, was the sex object.

I suppose the human race is doing the best it can under the circumstances, but hell's bells, that's only an explanation, not an excuse.

Lesson: Italy is a different country. They do things differently there.

Tableau Three:

Two Very Sick People and One Not-as-Sick Administrator

Baylor College of Medicine
Patients Ruth Hylbak, Penny Bailey, and a Medicare Administrator

Gertrude had myasthenia, reminding me of some other patients with myasthenia, many of whom were very sick. For instance, Ruth Hylbak spent months on a respirator. She became unable to chew, swallow, or talk. Soon thereafter, she was unable to move a single muscle. People who came into her room saw a body lying there still as a stone except for the up and down chest movements caused by the respirator.

Ruth's disease did not respond to any of the usual treatments, so I decided to try an experiment. Myasthenia is caused by antibodies attacking the connection between the nerves and the muscles. So the treatments are directed against the antibodies that are attacking. Ruth had her thymus removed in the hope that would stop the antibodies. It did not. She had taken a host of medicines to stop antibody production. They didn't work either. In fact, there were no other known ways of hitting this disease. So what do you do if you don't know what to do? Answer: you analyze the situation and act accordingly.

The human spleen is a lymphoid organ harboring antibody-producing cells, so I decided it might be a good idea to remove Ruth's spleen to see what would happen. No committees were involved in this decision. No permission was given by anyone to me to do or try such a thing. In those days, the doctor and the patient just decided what to do, and that was that.

The Doctor is in Charge

I was running the show. However, it would have been nice to get Ruth's permission. But Ruth was in no condition to give permission. She could not move a single muscle. The only way people knew she was alive was her pupils responded to light, and her heart was still beating.

Her mother: "Ruth wants you to do anything you want, but I can't give permission for the operation, because I don't want the responsibility."

"You're joking. You just told me Ruth wants me to do anything. You are just giving me the permission she gave you to give to me. You are her proxy. Ruth is giving permission through you."

Ruth's mother shook her head and started to cry. "I can't do it. If she dies, I would never forgive myself. You have to act on your own."

So, I guess, the removal of the spleen will proceed with a kind of informal verbal consent transferred from the patient to the patient's mother to me. At this time, Ruth herself is too sick to communicate anything. Informed consent, in this case, is impossible. Informed consent is overrated anyway. Is there such a thing? If someone told you everything that might happen when you drive your car to the movies, they would probably spend all day and all night and still not cover all the possible adverse events. In fact, informed consent or the attempt to get fully informed consent can have complications as severe as any medical treatment or operation. Two examples will appear in this narrative in due time.

Stanley Crawford, my surgeon friend, agreed to remove the spleen on my say-so, but when he and his resident visited the room, they thought Ruth was already dead. Imagine how frightening it must have been for poor Ruth to have some surgeons hovering over her and saying absurd things like, "This patient is dead. Bernie must not know she's dead."

Stanley and his resident were surprised when I showed them Ruth's pupils contracted to light.

"She is alive all right, just in very bad shape. "Ruth," I shouted. "Don't pay any attention to these jerks. They are surgeons. They don't know anything about myasthenia."

Stanley chimed in, "I don't even know how to say it, much less what it's about. But, if Bernie wants your spleen out, we can do that—no question."

"Ruth, I want them to cut out your spleen because I think that will help. There is some evidence, well not really evidence, conjecture really, my idea really, that the spleen has cells in it making antibodies that are making you weak. So, taking out your spleen should help, and if it doesn't, we'll try something else. OK? And if that doesn't work, we will try something else. We'll keep trying. We will never give up. I will never give up. OK? Ruth, I know you can't tell me yes or no, so I am assuming you would say yes if you could say something. Tomorrow, they will take you to the operating room, and I will stand by to make sure you are OK before, during, and after the operation. I am not worried about you. You are strong in spirit. You will survive this illness. You will get back in shape by sheer strength of will and the power of my medicine."

Notice, even when the condition is perilous, I focus on encouraging elements by indulging in pollyannish cant. Faith and optimism have life-giving qualities. Some patients recover health just on faith in the doctor. Faith comes from trust and is a critical aspect of healing. Optimism is a Patten moral imperative and, for the physician whose role is to affirm life, a medical imperative. Even when the outlook is grim, affirmative action and words promote well-being and shift the odds in favor of recovery.

The major problem in the present litigious age is an innovative approach can fail, and the consequences are likely to be far worse if the procedure is novel and untested or not approved. Fear of lawsuits makes physicians hesitant, circumspect, and as a result, often ineffective in cases where the patient is seriously ill and needs special innovative treatment.

The Danger

Operating on a myasthenic patient is hazardous, and operating on a patient like Ruth, who was in terrible shape, is even more hazardous. In the operating room, the bravest person would, of course, be Ruth. But what would you do? Sometimes a cliché is essential in understanding my vision: I had to carry the fight within the jaws of death itself. It was either continue to fight or give up. Tell me, did I do the right thing? Would you in my place have removed Ruth's spleen on the outside chance removal would solve her problem? Would you have dared? Would you have had the guts? Would you have acted without any formal legal permission?

I pause for reply.

Let us ask. What is the social value of a pain eased? What is the value of a life saved? How does the cure of a serious disease compare in value to a well-paved highway? How does making a complex diagnosis compare with flying a UTA jet plane to Papeete? You cannot say or guess. For you don't know. The comparative method is absurd. To think too much is to think too much. You cannot expect to measure the value of Ruth's life as though it were stock in a warehouse. My job was to help her survive, and, by God, that is what I would do and do it NOT AS A STRANGER. If our situations were reversed and Ruth was my doctor and I her patient, I would want Ruth to take out my spleen as a last-ditch desperate effort to cure my disease. Furthermore, if Ruth were my doctor, I would want her to treat me as I was treating her: not as a stranger, but as a friend.

What Happened?
Next Day. Ruth is Post-Op.

Ruth's mother met me outside the operating room.

"How is she?" she asked.

"I'm encouraged," I said positively gleeful.

"Why?"

"Well, for one thing, she's still alive! That's a miracle. And the spleen is out. It was larger than normal. The surgeons have removed several billion of the cells making Ruth sick."

"Will she recover?"

"I hope so. But I don't know. I don't have a crystal ball. I can't predict the future."

Result

Two weeks after the spleen had been removed, Ruth was able to breathe on her own, and two weeks after, she was walking and talking. Ruth spent decades as a painter of beautiful pictures and made her living as a commercial artist. She is the star of the movie we made for the Myasthenia Foundation. The movie, titled "New Hope" was, and may still be, the official film for lay people about myasthenia gravis. Ruth is also the star of the official movie of the Myasthenia Foundation for the instruction of physicians and the United States Department of Defense. The film is entitled "Diagnosis and Treatment of Myasthenia Gravis."

After her recovery, Ruth painted a portrait of how she remembered I looked when I told her about the spleen operation (photo).

Of course, this miracle of Ruth's spectacular recovery could not have happened without Stanley Crawford and his superb surgery. Once a patient said to Stanley, "Doctor Crawford, I can tell by the way you talk, you don't believe in God." Stanley smiled and said, "I beg your pardon, madam, I am God." Truth to tell, that is the way he and some of the other surgeons at Methodist Hospital viewed themselves. And why not? To do what they did and do, you had to have a gigantic ego and supreme confidence in yourself. There were giants in the earth in the old days, and Stanley Crawford was one of them.

About Stanley Crawford

When I first arrived in Houston in 1973, I called Stanley Crawford and asked him to find out for me who was the best surgeon to do thymectomies (removal of thymus) for my myasthenic patients. He said, "I'll check around and call you back." Nine minutes later, Stanley was back on the phone, "I checked. The best surgeon is ME!"

Penny Bailey—Another Very Sick Person

Penny was almost as sick as Ruth and spent months in the intensive care unit on a respirator. The new philosophy about conserving medical resources was beginning to take hold. There was pressure on me from the nurses, the residents, and some of my fellow attending neurologists: "Give up on Penny. Just let her go."

My resident, André, told me off in no uncertain terms: "She will never recover. You are beating a dead horse. You are wasting time and medical resources. Her case is hopeless. Let her go."

"André, I hope to hell she recovers, and when she does it will be one of the most important lessons you will ever learn about myasthenia gravis. The disease is treatable. Recovery is always possible, even in the sickest patient. In myasthenia, we never give up. We just have to find the key to liberate her from the disease."

The hospital administration also wanted the supposed waste to stop. Why they did I don't know. I would have thought the longer the patient stayed, the more the hospital got paid. Now I know that is not true. The less the stay, the more the pay, and the reason there is such a gigantic thrust to discharge patients. Evidently, hospitals get paid by diagnosis and not so much by length of stay. But I didn't know what the exact situation was with the hospital at the time, and I didn't care. I still don't know, and I still don't care. The Methodist Hospital had plenty of money for lavish parties and great pay for administrators. The hospital could handle the costs of taking care of a hundred Penny Baileys. Although not for profit, hospitals are really big businesses.

Support from Clergy

Major support for keeping up the treatments on Penny came from the chaplains of the Methodist Hospital, not only the Catholic chaplain, but also the Rabbi and the Methodist chaplain. They were behind me 100% and spoke in my favor multiple times. Religion does have redeeming features. This was a big one for me and a very big one for Penny. Many thanks, chaplains. You helped protect the vulnerable, the sick, the weak, the defenseless. If you don't mind my saying so, it was a real Christian thing to do. Many thanks.

Every day on rounds, Penny wrote on a slate: "When will I get off the respirator?" And every day she got the same answer from me: "How should I know? I don't have a crystal ball."

(Note: crystal ball is an ancient medical device used to see into the future and thereby predict a patient's future and prognosis.)

Result

With time and the proper treatments, Penny made a great recovery and became, for a time, a fashion model.

Luisa Markowsky, the head clinical nurse for my practice, and I attended a big celebration in Penny's hometown, Dyersburg, Tennessee. The mayor of that fair city, Penny's father, gave me the key to the city (see letter from Hester and Richard Hill, Penny's parents).

The Dyersburg key is the biggest and the most valuable of all the city keys in my collection of five, but the key to Corpus Christi, Texas, though smaller, is the most colorful.

Penny herself gave me a crystal ball and told me, "Never again will you be able to tell patients you don't have a crystal ball."

She is right. From that day forward, I never told any patient I didn't have a crystal ball. Instead, I would tell them, "I have a crystal ball. But it is not working, so I can't predict the future."

Citizens of Dyersburg chipped in to pay Penny's hospital bill. That was nice of them and nice for the Methodist Hospital.

Coda

Myasthenia is a treatable disease. All you have to do is find the treatment that works in that individual patient. The trouble is sometimes finding the correct treatment requires time, energy, and money. Sometimes it requires lots of time, energy, and money and, more importantly, deep critical thinking. It doesn't just happen. You have to work at it.

> **Lesson:** Arguments about conserving medical resources are weak arguments.

Next time you hear arguments about wasting medical resources, think about Ruth and Penny and look at who's talking. Chances are the person who is talking is healthy, and chances are the person they want deprived is too sick to defend herself and her interests. Thus, there is a kind of exploitation of the sick.

This argument, their arguments, of course, fell on my deaf ears, but so what? It did not matter, for the situation in those days was the physician in charge was in charge, like the captain of a ship. They could try to get me to change course, but they couldn't make me.

Nowadays, things have changed. Now the insurance company says, "You can do what you want, but we won't pay for it, and you won't be paid."

Lesson: Complex situations cannot be governed by simple rules.

The fundamental problem is the misguided perspective that health care is a binary world in which interventions are either effective or not effective, appropriate or inappropriate. The truth is there are lots of gray zones in which the care is neither clearly justified or not clearly justified—zones whose benefits are unknown or uncertain and whose value may depend on the patient's preference and the available alternatives. Gray zones are the rule when we deal with previously unrecognized diseases, new treatments, or new techniques. One of the first lawsuits I won involved the use of Magnetic Resonance Imaging (MRI) in a patient suspected of having multiple sclerosis. The insurance carrier did not pay the 800-some-odd dollars for this test because they believed it was "unapproved" and "medically unnecessary." At the time, MRI was unapproved and just coming into its own, so I understood the insurance company's position.

Except, they were wrong.

Now, every reasonable neurologist would agree with me and the judge on this case who said, "The doctor, not a company, should be making the decisions about what is or what is not needed." Thus, MRI for diagnosis and appraisal of multiple sclerosis used to be in the gray zone. No more. Now MRI is used in multiple sclerosis to show the extent and the activity of the disease and help determine the best treatments for a particular patient at a particular time. company

The result of that lawsuit taught me a lesson. So instead of just saluting when the insurance said they wouldn't pay, I sued them acting as my own attorney. I won 44 cases and lost one against Blue Cross and Blue Shield of Texas who said my admission of an old women with a stroke and high blood pressure was not necessary. The patient, now fully recovered, testified to the contrary, but the judge would not admit her testimony because he thought the patient's opinion was irrelevant. My six-page appeal to the three-judge appeal court in Washington, D.C. resulted in a reversal of the trial judge's decision and an order in my favor. Blue Cross and Blue Shield had to eat crow. They paid the bills, and they paid me, and they paid me interest.

The Director of Medicare Lectures Me

About this same topic: the regional director of Medicare told me I should not have admitted an old man (he was 82) to the hospital because he went blind in one eye. According to her: "Blindness in one eye is not serious and can be managed in an outpatient setting."

How did I answer her? The patient in question had temporal arteritis and went blind in his right eye. He came to the emergency room because the vision in the left eye was failing. This situation is well known as a cause of blindness, and I gave an intravenous injection of hydrocortisone within five minutes of seeing the patient. That treatment is effective and saved his vision in the left eye. He was admitted to try to restore vision in the right eye. But once the vision goes out in this disease, the chance of reversal is slim. He remained blind in the right eye despite the treatments. The patient was happy, even if Medicare was not going to pay for his admission. "In the kingdom of the blind, the one-eyed man is king" to quote a famous book by H.G. Wells.

And besides, my 82-year-old patient owned a bank chain in Texas, so he could, and would pay even if Medicare didn't.

But, you know, this situation set me to thinking I should avoid the bullshit and drop out of Medicare.

To the director of Medicare, what were my arguments?

Moral argument: this mode of handling patients is a part of the whole system of fraud and inhumanity. The sick person paid insurance premiums for decades and paid Medicare taxes for decades. Now that it is time to get something back for all those payments and all the promises of help and succorance, there is talk of cutting back and reneging on the obligations promised. Not fair or just! It is a violation of contract.

"Vengeance is Mine," Says the Lord

Does a righteous God govern the universe? And for what does he hold the lightning bolts in his right hand, if not to smite the oppressor and deliver the sick out of the hands of the spoiler?

Or is there really a goddess named Fortuna who seeks to show us mortals the force of fate and the power of destiny? Who knows? What I do know is within two weeks the Medicare administrator, the same who lectured me about how to take care of the old man who went blind in one eye, lost vision in her right eye. She called me and asked to be admitted to the hospital as an emergency!

I took care of her, of course, without reprimand. She was sick and needed help.

I fiddled with my ophthalmoscope, adjusting the lens dial, put my face close up to hers, and focused on her optic nerve. Poets tell us eyes are the windows to the soul. They are also the windows to the brain. Examining the back of the eye gives a pretty good idea about the state of the brain, as you will see in several cases that follow.

Her vision was extinguished by a small piece of cholesterol plaque broken off from an atherosclerotic ulcer in her right carotid artery. These emboli, seen with the ophthalmoscope, cause transient loss of vision in the medical condition known as amaurosis fugax (Latin: fleeting blindness).

Most times, the embolus passes forward and the blindness remits. In this case, the embolus was still there, but by using pressure on the orbital globe, I was able to dislodge the embolus, and my patient's vision returned as the blood flow returned. It returned to 20/40, not the 20/20 she had had prior to the event. The amaurosis fugax is a transient ischemic attack that may be the harbinger of a future stroke. So, knowing that, what would you do to prevent a stroke? What should be done? The question bugged me for two weeks.

Yes, I kept her in the hospital while I tried to think about the best way to handle the patient's problem. Once, I kept a patient in for six weeks while I tried to decide if the patient needed a myelogram and back surgery. He did. Doing surgery is the easy part. Deciding if the patient needs surgery is the hard part. Usually, if a patient with a severe back problem has not improved after six weeks of rest and medicines, surgery is the way to go.

All things considered, I advised our Director of Medicare to have a surgical removal of the atherosclerotic plaque in her carotid artery, and she agreed. My patient left the hospital a happier and wiser person and with a much better chance of not having a major stroke in the distribution of her right carotid artery.

Right to Life is Still a Fight as Reported in the Houston Chronicle, Section B, Page One, Article by Dylan Baddoue, Friday, December 18, 2015

Texas Right to Life has sued Houston Methodist Hospital on behalf of Chris Dunn, 46, after a hospital committee determined that further efforts to sustain Dunn's life would only prolong his suffering. The organization wants the hospital to keep Dunn on a breathing machine and to provide additional medical care. Texas Right to Life has taken up the cause of some 300 patients in similar situations. But Dunn is the first case in which the patient and family were willing to share the story publicly and the patient was alert enough to make his wishes known in a video, which has caught the attention of conservative websites and others online. Dunn wants to live, doesn't mind the suffering, and wants full care. I would too because I think once I would be dead there would be no coming back. I would be dead for a long, long time. Probably billions of years. Other people would have a different view of this issue. How about you?

Who Decides?

So, the question in the Dunn case is who the decider is. Who decides when care should be stopped? The hospital? Some committee? The doctors? The patient? The family? Who?

Does the patient have a right to dictate how much care he gets or does a hospital committee? Evelyn Kelly, Dunn's mother, said of her son's illness, "He's too young to die." Kelly said she believes the decision was based on her son's lack of insurance and inability to pay for his care. Stefanie Asin, a Houston Methodist spokeswoman, said this was untrue, noting the hospital's $126 million annual charity care budget. "This has absolutely nothing to do with insurance," Asin said.

Note: Houston Methodist does have a $126 million annual charity care budget. But it would be interesting to know how much of is actually spent on charity care. When I was attending neurologist there, the answer was "not much."

Result

The courts disagreed with the hospital and the hospital's committee. A judge twice blocked termination of Dunn's treatment. The judge felt the patient was more qualified to decide if he wanted to live or not.

Good!

What is unique about Chris Dunn's case is that Dunn wanted to live and was alive enough to express his wish that all care be continued including the respirator. Other patients are not so fortunate. They are unconscious and not able to contradict the opinions of the hospitals who want to get rid of them.

Methodist obeyed the court and continued care until Dunn died of "natural causes" just a few weeks after his YouTube video (wherein he begged for his life) went viral.

Thus, Chris Dunn, a patient with no insurance taken care of at Methodist Hospital for two months, a former police officer, a former Homeland Security officer, a former EMT, died at age 46 while on the respirator. His family, in a public statement, agreed he died of "natural causes" and that Methodist continued care until Dunn's death. What these "natural causes" were was never revealed either by the family or by the hospital.

Craig Goes Blind

Talking about blindness reminds me of when my son, Craig, lost his vision. He was in the third grade at the time, so he must have been eight years old. One Sunday night, while I was kissing him goodnight, he said, "Dad, does it mean anything when you can't see out of your left eye?"

"What do you mean?"

"My left eye clouded over."

"Close your right eye and count the fingers I hold in front of your face."

"I can't see any fingers."

I called Bob Zeller, the best pediatric neurologist in Houston. "Bob, meet me in the ER. Craig lost his vision in the left eye."

There followed a frantic drive to the Texas Children's Hospital. Craig was in the back seat. Halfway there, he says, "The same thing is happening with my right eye. I can't see the moon anymore. Do you think this will affect my career as an airplane pilot?"

Bob Zeller met us at the hospital, admitted Craig, and started intravenous corticosteroids for optic neuritis. I slept in a chair in Craig's room during the two anxious weeks he was a patient. I held him down during the spinal tap, and I learned how important the medical mission could be. And I learned the hard way the last thing you get in a hospital is peace, rest, quiet, or a good night's sleep.

Bob Zeller, who was one of my junior residents when I was the chief resident at Columbia, was now like a god. Craig and I waited for Bob to round in the afternoons. We hung on Bob's every word, and we appreciated his caring for us as friends and not as strangers. The treatments worked. Craig recovered. He never became a pilot, but he did get a Ph.D. in biophysics.

Tableau Four:

A Grandmother Who Went Into a Coma While Playing Bridge and a Socialite Who is Proud of the Disease She Had

A Grandmother Who Went Into a Coma While Playing Bridge and a Socialite

Baylor College of Medicine

Talking about the emergency room reminded me of an elderly woman who, at a tournament at the Shamrock Hilton Hotel in Houston, collapsed while playing bridge. It was the third day of the tournament when she dropped her hand and fell face forward flat onto the card table. They rushed her to the emergency room of the Methodist Hospital, where, on examination, she was in a coma with no responses to any stimulus, including pinching, jabbing with a needle, loud shouting, and so forth. Her pupils were dilated and did not respond to light. The Glasgow Coma Scale was 3, severe—the lowest you can go. The nurse on duty said, "She's finished. No sense wasting time. Probably had a cerebral hemorrhage or brain stem (infarction) or a cardiac arrest. Anyway, she's brain dead."

"You're probably right," I said as I drew blood for everything I could think of. "But nurse, go fetch a 50cc syringe with 50% glucose for intravenous injection. She might be hypoglycemic (low blood sugar). We don't want her to die of something stupid." Inject glucose is what I always do on the outside chance this kind of patient is suffering from low blood sugar as the cause of the coma.

Result

Bingo! She awoke! Dazed. She looks around. "Where am I?"

About 10 minutes later, the laboratory reported a blood sugar of 18! A coma level of blood sugar explains the coma.

But what explains the low blood sugar? Aye, that's the question. Always try to get to the bottom of things. It requires a little more effort but sometimes does show the complexity surrounding the human situation.

The answer: playing Sherlock Holmes, I went to the pharmacy and inspected the written prescription. Our patient arrived at the Shamrock hotel with a sore throat and consulted the hotel doctor who prescribed an antibiotic, Aureomycin (chlortetracycline). That was a good bet for a sore throat. It is a broad spectrum antibiotic and should clear up the sore throat if the sore throat were due to a bacterial organism sensitive to the antibiotic. But the pharmacist, misreading the doctor's miserable handwriting, dispensed acetohexamide (Dymelor), a first-generation sulfonylurea that is used to treat type 2 diabetes. Acetohexamide lowers blood sugar by stimulating the pancreas to secrete insulin. The pancreas is needed for acetohexamide to work, and that's the reason this medicine is not used in type 1 diabetes where the insulin-secreting cells are no longer working.

So, for three days, four times a day, she took a drug that lowers blood sugar and wondered why her sore throat did not improve. And no, she did not sue the pharmacist or the doctor or the hotel. She was just grateful to be alive and back to her old self and able to play bridge. And think about this: if she had not received the glucose, she would have died, and the autopsy would have shown, as a cause of death—ABSOLUTELY NOTHING.

Socialite Y
Baylor College of Medicine

She was 82 and in excellent health until about three months ago when she developed severe headaches, stiff neck, blurred vision, decreased attention span, and poor memory. Her record as a major contributor to the social scene in this fair city and her multiple charities, which included a gigantic donation to the medical school and to the medical center, made me proud she selected me to take care of her. It was an honor and a privilege.

Examination showed a lively, happy, charming woman who had a stiff neck in all positions, severe papilledema (meaning there was marked increase in intracranial pressure), and some difficulty, but not much, with the routine tests of memory.

Conclusion: she had chronic meningitis. During the year, I had seen three cases due to yeast meningitis. I thought this was another case.

To get at the cause, a spinal tap needed to be done and in view of her social position, I decided to do it myself. The measured opening pressure was, as expected, very high and the fluid was slightly yellow. As I collected multiple tubes of spinal fluid something extraordinary happened: the fluid clotted! This meant the protein content of the spinal fluid was very high, and the protein had denatured as it came out of the needle into the tube. Denatured proteins are what cause egg albumin to clot when heated or cream to become semisolid when whipped. During my sub-internship at Belleview Hospital (New York City) there were patients who had chronic meningitis and clotted spinal fluid. All those patients had syphilis, so I assumed Patient Y had syphilis too. No need to tell her until the lab confirms the diagnosis. When she learns the truth, drama is expected. Most patients are not happy when they are told they have syphilis, or AIDS, or cancer, or leprosy, or multiple sclerosis, or sphingomyelia, and so forth, but they must be told. And the doctor is the person to tell them. Right?

Mrs. Y came with me to the treatment room for a private talk. I closed and locked the door. We are alone. No one can overhear what I was about to say. No one can overhear this deep dark secret.

A Grandmother Who Went Into a Coma While Playing Bridge and a Socialite

She: "What's up Doc? Why the hush-hush?"

Me: "Sally, the good news is we have a definite diagnosis. The disease you have is very treatable. The most likely outcome is you will be cured."

She: "Thank, God! I was afraid I had old timer's disease.

Me: "Nope, Sally, you do not have Alzheimer's disease.

She: "So? What do I have?

Me: "You have chronic meningitis due to syphilis."

She: "Syphilis? You mean the sex disease? Syphilis caused the headaches, lights bothering my eyes, the blurred vision? Syphilis is making me feel like a sicko?"

Me: "Yep. Syphilis is the great imitator and can simulate almost any nervous system condition. In you, it produced chronic infection and inflammation of the coverings of the brain. The organism is sensitive to antibiotics, particularly penicillin, so we are going to kill the bug that is trying to kill you."

Socialite Y jumps off the treatment table, smiles, hugs me, and gives me a big wet kiss on the right cheek. She steps back.

She: "Wow! Syphilis! I'm not surprised. In my salad days I was wild. Real wild."

Me: "That's the good news. The bad news is all venereal diseases, except AIDS, must be reported. The public health nurse will soon be knocking on your door to ask about your sex life. Understand?"

She: "Oh yes, Doctor. Of course! I wouldn't wish trouble on any of my men friends. Let's get to the bottom of it. Treat them if they need treatment. But we have to be discrete. You know what I mean?"

Me: "Some are married?"

She: "Yes. Some are married. Some are not. Some are young and some are not so young. The only one not married is me. My husband died ages ago and is now enjoying his eternal reward. No problem with him. But there will be stormy weather among some of the wives. Syphilis is not my real problem. It is merely the consequence of my real problem"

Me: "Your real problem?"

She: "The trouble started as a teenager. I worshipped boys, and then I worshipped men. I still do, but not as much as then. When I look at a man, I don't see a human being. I see a god, an Adonis. To me men are the most delicious thing on this planet. It is a personal failing. I can't help it. I love them, and I will love them until I die. And I love what they do to me, and I love how they make me feel, and I love how they smell and how they taste. I love everything about them."

Me: "Very interesting. Same thing with me. Only in reverse. I don't see women. I see goddesses. I hope sometime to be able to see them as humans. It is really hard. To me, women are the most beautiful thing in the world. And men are low down, dirty, and deceptive. That the goddesses, like you, would have anything to do with men puzzles me. But they do. To each his own and nature's way."

Result: Complete Cure after Penicillin Rx.

None of Y's sexual contacts tested positive for syphilis, so wives were not bothered about the situation. Where she originally got the disease is a mystery to her and to us, her physicians (two infectious disease experts were consulted about what treatment was best).

Six of her sexual contacts were dead, so the public health nurse will not be talking to them. Perhaps one of them was the culprit. Late-stage syphilis meningitis is not contagious, so Y could not recently infect anyone. After treatment, she was disease-free and, unless reinfected, unable to spread the disease.

Her beauty, though faded, still attracts men (including me). I saw her dining with a handsome elderly fellow at Charley's 517 here in Houston. They toasted martinis together and gave each other "that look." Naturally, I did not say hello.

Of the divine nature of women, I have no doubt. Of their animal nature, I have no doubt.

* * *

Sidebar about Insurance People Telling Doctors
What to Do and What Not to Do

Getting talked to by a mere administrator was an earthquake to me. She was advising me on how to manage a patient's illness, and yet she had not seen the patient.

A Grandmother Who Went Into a Coma While Playing Bridge and a Socialite

She did not get a history or do a physical examination. She did not do a neurological examination, and more important, she had not suffered through four years of medical school, a rough year of internship, three years of neurology residency, a year of memory fellowship, and two years of neuromuscular disease fellowship. God only knew how many patients she had taken care of who had lost vision in an eye. Not a single one, I would bet, else she would have been practicing medicine without a license. Few could match my experience in the medical realm. Yet, she felt qualified to tell me what to do! The situation was and is absurd. Talk to any practicing physician at the next cocktail party about this and the daily inconveniences and irritations of their professional life.

Some of their grievances are real enough. The general tone is resentment at the felt and not-quite-understood fact that the ancient status of the medical profession is now obsolete. In fact, I have a feeling most physicians are burned out. I know a 2016 survey conducted by the American Academy of Neurology proved, in fact, most neurologists consider themselves burned out and are in general dissatisfied with their lifestyle.

Time marches on, and administrators and insurance companies have taken over. They have the power, and physicians must bow to them to get paid. Doctors brought this on themselves by being so obedient to power and saluting at every damn thing that came down the pike even if that damn thing was contrary to the doctor's interest, or the patients' interest, or both. The trouble was, and is, doctors went to medical school where they learned to take orders without question. Doctors have been culturally conditioned not to fight back. Too bad!

The debate about Obamacare rationing medical care was a joke. Medical care is already rationed by corporate America and corporate greed. In my view, insurance companies are responsible for barriers to health care and for excess administrative waste. Concerned with maintaining profit margins, insurance companies limit access for covered care through high deductibles and gatekeepers. They attempted to obstruct care by policies that excluded preexisting conditions and lifetime limits. Payers have created mountains of red tape with inefficiencies in billing and coding without any benefits to quality of care or health outcomes. Therefore, corporate practice of medicine = insane.

My daughter Allegra, who is a neurologist, tells me now doctors must receive permission to order tests, scans, and x-rays. That's absurd. Allegra says the insurance company can even substitute for a prescription drug another drug they think will be effective but costs less. They call it the step-up program. The patient must take the less expensive (and often less effective medicine) first, and then, and only then, can they step up to the better more effective and more expensive treatment. Absurd, right? Needless to say, some patients die before they get the opportunity to step up!

At my medical school's 25th reunion (1991), in general my classmates were happy. But there was an underlying current of discontent, disappointment, and demoralization because of what medical practice was becoming. The complaints are both financial and vocational. Insurance pay is usually slow, low, or no pay. Compounding the pay problem is the loss of autonomy, authority, and respect. Doctors are now providers, not physicians. There seems to be a never-ending attack on the profession by government, insurance companies, and lawyers. A major problem is unproductive rules and regulations topped by an electric medical record system designed to provide billing information and not to advance patient care. I have seen them already—print outs handed to patients from their electronic medical record. They are loaded with bilge—most of it inaccurate and some of it just wrong. Ethel's print out stated she had cystic fibrosis, instead of polycystic breasts! No patient with cystic fibrosis would be alive at her age. It took her several hours to correct the mistake. Checkboxes, templates, copy and paste might look good for the bill to the insurance company, but is of little scientific or epidemiological utility and interferes with the clinician's work.

All this stuff takes its toll on the doctor's time and energy and wastes an important national resource. My urologist recently told me that he feels he is just a highly paid data entry clerk.

But there is balm in Gilead. At my school's 50th reunion most of my classmates were happy. Many of them had left medicine and were retired or in business or had gone to law school and were now practicing law. Some had become writers like Robin Cook and yours truly.

The Theory of Metasynthetic Wisdom and Open Giant Complex Systems

The human mind has trouble understanding the vast complexity of the real world. Reductionist thinking, which breaks down complex systems into smaller more easily managed parts, seems to be the easier way for us to grasp our environment and to understand medical problems. That paradigm gets us only so far and is unsuitable for managing complex systems existing in a sick patient. Clinical medicine requires, I firmly believe, a different approach than the application of reductionist analysis. No simple cookbook or set of guidelines can possibly encompass the complexity of dealing with individual patients and their illness. Thus, medicine must remain an art and a science, and the doctors must exert a human understanding of each individual patient to obtain the best results. Do you agree?

Jackson G. Smith Gets Revenge on His Insurance Company and Stephen Hawking Decides He Doesn't Want to be Treated for His Condition

Baylor College of Medicine

My patient Jackson G. Smith had fun. He was diagnosed in 1987 by a Birmingham, Alabama doctor as having amyotrophic lateral sclerosis (ALS). This is a fatal disease and there was no treatment for it. Jackson decided to read up on his disease, and he found my article about ALS being a syndrome, a running together of signs and symptoms. My article advised complete and detailed study of individual patients in the hope of finding they had something that looked like ALS but was not ALS. Bingo! Jackson had a demyelinating neuropathy, and not ALS. Severe cases of this disease have been mistaken for ALS, and one very famous mathematician in England probably had been misdiagnosed as well. His name is Stephen Hawking. You will soon read about his case and my dinner with him in London. Meanwhile, let's get back to patient Jackson.

I treated Jackson, a 41-year-old roofer, with Cytoxan, a very powerful immunosuppressant drug used in chemotherapy, and he improved. Then in 1990, because he was still very weak, I prescribed intravenous gamma globulin. His Milwaukee-based insurance company, Time Insurance, Inc., paid for the chemotherapy but balked at the gamma globulin treatment, mainly because it was so expensive. But, of course, they did not cite the expense as the reason they refused to pay. Instead, they said the gamma globulin "was experimental and not medically necessary." And in a way, it was experimental. Every time you give a patient a treatment, you are experimenting to see what will happen. As every patient is unique, medical work is essentially experimental, uncertain, and, consequently, prone to error. And no treatment is absolutely necessary. The law requires we cover our nudity, and that can be done with newspaper. Thus, strictly speaking, shirts, dresses, shoes, socks, and so forth are not necessary. Get it? The not necessary thing is a fiction designed to swell bottom line profits for the insurance company. The truth is: no treatment is absolutely necessary. We can always just let the disease continue and not do anything. Some patients may recover. Some will not recover. Some will get worse as the disease progresses. Some will die. Whatever happens with the neglect will be good for the insurance company and perhaps not so good for the insured.

Lesson: Be aware of diversionary arguments when money is involved. Those arguments are designed to focus your attention away from the real issue on to something fake. When an insurance company claims a medical treatment is not necessary, the real reason they say or think that may be they don't want to pay, and they don't want to pay because they want to increase profits.

Result: Because His Insurance Company Refused to Pay for His Treatment, Patient Jackson Himself Paid. Hooray for Jackson!

Yes, Jackson, now 47 years old, footed the bill for the gamma globulin and recovered his health. Yes, you read correctly. Jackson became normal. Now Time Insurance was in trouble because the treatment they said was not necessary had worked and restored Jackson to normal functioning. Yes, that is not a misprint. He was normal and now back to work roofing and mighty mad about what had happened. Jackson felt his insurance company had screwed him. So, in the great American tradition, Jackson sued his insurance company.

The Federal Court jury, following a five-day trial before Senior U.S. District Court Judge Virgil Pittman, awarded Jackson the $10,000 cost of the gamma globulin and gave him $1,250,000 for mental anguish and an additional $3,500,000 punitive damages (see newspaper story among pictures and documents).

Gamma globulin is now a routine treatment for demyelinating neuropathy and has restored many patients to health. The companies pay for it, and so does Medicare. They have to. Or at least they had to for a time, until the insurance companies invented the step-up system. Now patients have to take the less expensive treatment first, and if it doesn't work, then, and only then, can they step up to the more expensive treatment. Meanwhile, patients waiting to step up have to suffer, and some have to die.

> **Lesson:** The step-up system requires the treatment receive prior approval from the insurance company. The cheapest treatment must be applied first, and then, if and only if it fails, will the more expensive "stepped up" treatment be approved. In general, this is a great idea if you wish to limit the freedom of patients and doctors to choose their treatment and a great idea to improve insurance company profits.

As for me, if I were sick, I would want the most effective treatment first, and I definitely want the same for my patients. How about you? Not every patient can wait to go through the steps. And there is always the problem of the disease killing them before they get to the effective next step.

> **Lesson:** Don't step up.

Jackson G. Smith Gets Revenge on His Insurance Company

Result

The Jackson award is, according to Mark Spear, Jackson's attorney, one of the biggest bad faith verdicts ever rendered in the State of Alabama. Spear told Cathy Donelson, staff reporter for the Mobile Press (page 2B, Tuesday, December 1, 1992), the case involved two similar diseases. "Both were nerve diseases, but one is treatable and the other is not." That is indeed the crux of the matter.

Stephen Hawking

Courtesy of the London Medical Society, I lectured for four days in London on the topic amyotrophic lateral sclerosis. The schedule was lectures on Monday, Tuesday, Wednesday, then Thursday off, and the last day of lectures was on Friday.

Stephen Hawking, the Lucasian Professor of Mathematics at Cambridge, came to every lecture. He had been diagnosed as having ALS at age 21 and was given two years to live. He came to my lectures because he wanted to learn about his problem. He always arrived in a wheelchair with his nurse and stayed front row center right under my podium. He was a physical wreck—all crunched up and unable to talk, walk, or even adjust his position in the chair. His face was distorted and his lips everted, and he was drooling.

He was a physical wreck, but he was still carrying on. I would not in any way diminish his accomplishments and his courage. The world is a better place because of him. If you have time, take a look at the movie "The Theory of Everything" which shows the struggles, triumphs, successes, and failures of thousands of patients like him who manage to deal with gigantic handicaps and hardships and still maintain a joie de vivre. The lesson here is all lives count, especially to those who are living them even when they look wrecked.

Lesson: Most of us will, sooner or later, be made weak by time and fate. Therefore, make the most of your life right now and be prepared for a not-so-great future.

Be prepared. It is highly likely you and I, dear reader, will someday in the future have to step through the looking glass and be sick and weak and need help. We are all doomed. We are all suffering under a mysterious sentence of death. At age 100, I guarantee you will not look as good as you look now or be as fit. Your youth is your greatest weapon. Use it and your time wisely. Be intelligent. Be adventurous. Be all you can be.

As for me, I know I shall never be young again, but that fact does not prevent me from being immature.

Invitation

On Wednesday afternoon, his nurse handed me a note. It said: "Professor Hawking invites you to have dinner with him and his friends tonight."

I accepted.

The dinner took place at a private townhome. It was merry old England with stuffy chairs, servants in livery, a big library, and excellent roast beef with a nice claret from Bordeaux, France. Hawking's nurse fed him a white liquid via nasogastric tube. I tried to put some sugar on the situation by saying while the rest of us were eating roast beef, poor Stephen had to be content with what looked like white paint.

No response from Hawking, but the nurse laughed her head off. This was the same nurse who came with him to the lectures. It was clear to me she loved Hawking and I think he loved her back. Jane Wilde, who had married Hawking in 1965, did not attend the dinner.

The other people there were important, but at the time, in my vast ignorance, I didn't recognize their names. One of them was a Huxley, and one of them was a nice woman, named, I think, Dame Thorndike.

Hawking used a computer to speak. The program apologized for speaking American English, and not British English. It said it was an American program so American English was all it could speak. Hawking said, via the computer, in good idiomatic American, "My food is not white paint. It is ground up auto parts."

The next day I went with one of the women to Stonehenge, and on Friday I was back lecturing. Sometime Friday morning, the nurse handed me a note from Hawking saying he now realized that he didn't have ALS, and he would like to come to the United States to have me take care of him.

Arrangements were made, but he changed his mind. He decided that he was well adjusted to his disease and didn't want to change his situation. He knew now that his condition was not progressing (indeed he had been disabled much longer than the usual ALS patient lasts) so he was not so much worried about dying. And that was that. My take on the situation is he did the right thing because that is what he wanted.

But he also did the wrong thing in not giving himself a chance at recovery. Oh, well, we all make mistakes. He also made a big mistake when he said the Higgs Boson would never be discovered. It was.

To live over five decades with motor neuron disease would be quite unusual, but not impossible. The autopsy will tell the tale. In my view, he has a demyelination neuropathy, and I think he would have responded to treatment the way most patients do. Hawking has the same problem as Jackson—misdiagnosed as ALS, I believe, and would have probably had the same opposition to gamma globulin treatment and would have taken the treatment anyway and would have recovered as Jackson did. Medicine is not an exact science, but in some cases, like Jackson's case, it comes close. To his credit, Hawking, when asked about Trump, said, "He is a demagogue, who seems to appeal to the lowest common denominator."

Hawking was an atheist. He was quoted on BBC as saying, "God doesn't exist. No one directs our fate. There is no afterlife. No heaven and no hell. The universe came into existence by itself, created from nothing. We have this one life to appreciate the grand design of the universe, and for that I am extremely grateful."

In fact, this is not far off the scientific mark. Many subatomic particles come into existence all the time from nothing at all. Production of matter from nothing probably is a basic law of the universe just like gravity. And it is highly likely there is no heaven and no hell and no afterlife.

But the Hawking quote I like the best is what he said to Diane Sawyer of ABC News, June 2010: "There is a fundamental difference between religion, which is based on authority, (and) science, which is based on observation and reason. Science will win because it works."

Hawking and Jane campaigned for disability access and support at Cambridge. Later, he made strong statements supporting universal health care and stem cell research. He also called the U.S. invasion of Iraq a "war crime." He championed nuclear disarmament and supported strong efforts to address climate change. He said you are a fool if you don't believe in climate change. The real question is what is causing it and what can be done.

Living longer than expected, Hawking died at age 76 on March 14, 2018. His ashes are interred at Westminster Abbey near the graves of Isaac Newton and Charles Darwin.

Professor Hawking, a cripple in a wheelchair, reminds me of another cripple in a wheelchair—Andrew Brown. But first, a short introduction to help you handle Andrew's case.

Myasthenic Syndromes

Myasthenic syndromes, conditions which impair connections between nerve and muscle, include a congenital myasthenia due to defective release of transmitter from nerve to muscle, magnesium-related neuromuscular disease due to defective release of transmitter from nerve to muscle, the myasthenic syndrome of Eaton and Lambert due to defective release of transmitter from nerve to muscle (often associated with cancer of the lung), botulism due to defective release of transmitter from nerve to muscle, antibiotic and other drug-induced neuromuscular block due to defective release of transmitter from nerve to muscle, tick paralysis due to defective release of transmitter from nerve to muscle, scorpion sting and spider bite in secondary stage due to defective release of transmitter from nerve to muscle, ciguatera fish poisoning at least in part due to defective release of transmitter from nerve to muscle, blue-lipped octopus bite that blocks the sodium channel in the muscle preventing the muscle from contracting, paralytic shellfish poisoning due to saxitoxin which blocks the sodium channel like the octopus bite, and pufferfish poisoning where tetrodotoxin blocks the sodium channel and prevents muscle contraction.

The Kid from Canada Who Couldn't Walk

Patient Andrew Brown

Little eight-year-old Andrew Brown had been unable to walk his entire life and was wheelchair bound when he arrived at the hospital. Andrew was born with a rare disorder called congenital myasthenia gravis in which muscles are unable to receive messages from the brain due to a block of transmission at the junction of nerve to muscle.

"He spent his life in a wheelchair, in bed, or trying to push himself around in a walker," said Doug Brown, 36, of Toronto, Canada. Even more heartbreaking, Doug and his wife Mary, 34, lost a child to the same disease, congenital myasthenia, three years before Andrew was born.

Andrew's devoted parents took Andrew to the top specialists in their country and in the United States—but came up empty. Even the world's expert in congenital myasthenia, the doctor who discovered some of the exact mechanisms of muscular weakness in the condition, Andrew Engel, of Mayo Clinic, could not help.

Then they heard about a certain Doctor Patten who seemed to know things about myasthenia and they decided to give Doctor Patten a try.

So Mary stayed home with their three other children and Doug brought Andrew to Houston to see Doctor Patten at The Methodist Hospital.

I subjected Andrew to every test I could think of that might have some influence on muscle function. Andrew had pretty severe deficiencies in multiple vitamins and minerals because he had such great difficulty swallowing. Replacement would help set the stage for recovery of muscle function if the key defect in transmission could be corrected. One thing for sure: Andrew was severely deficient in iron and had a bad iron deficiency anemia. Correction of those problems made him feel better but had no direct effect on muscle weakness.

Something interesting about Andrew—he liked magic. On rounds, I did magic tricks for him. When he went to magnetic scan, he did not lie still, so the radiologist asked me if it were OK to put Andrew under general anesthesia to get the scan done. General anesthesia is a lot to handle for a myasthenic kid, and so I vetoed the idea. Instead, Andrew and I made a deal—if he kept still throughout the entire scan, I would teach him a magic trick. Nurses and other doctors were underwhelmed by this idea, and so was the radiologist. But what could they do? I was the physician in charge. What I say goes.

Andrew proved them wrong. Andrew stayed "still as a stone" according to the radiologist and earned his magic trick. I showed him how to pass a nickel through a rubber barrier and into a glass jar. With a few practices, Andrew could do the trick like a pro.

Speaking of tricks: an old trick in myasthenia gravis is to give ephedrine (in those days used for asthma relief) to increase the release of transmitter from the nerve to the muscle. Ephedrine was to be my main treatment. Notice the main treatment was withheld until everything correctable was corrected. Only then would we know for sure that if the ephedrine didn't work, it was because it didn't work and not because of some other confounding stupid thing like iron deficiency anemia or vitamin deficiency.

Result

"He swallowed it at 6 p.m.," said his father, Doug. "At 7 p.m., he started getting restless."

"Although Andrew couldn't walk, I had always let him out of bed at home and stand with me, so he could stretch as I held him. That evening, I asked, 'Do you want to stretch?'"

"Andrew said, 'Sure.' He swung his legs over the side of the bed, grabbed me, and stood up. Then a miracle happened—he pushed me away and started to walk. He was very unsteady, but he took one step, then another and another."

"I was astonished. I blurted, 'Andrew, you can walk!' He didn't say a word. He was concentrating everything on getting one foot in front of the other."

"I took his arm and incredibly, he walked to the nurses' station. A nurse started to cry. Tears were also streaming down my face."

"Then Andrew said, 'I don't believe this' and after that I couldn't get him to stop walking until finally, I persuaded him to get back to his hospital room."

The next day, after another dose of medicine, Andrew was up again and walking. Three days later, Doug used Andrew's wheelchair to carry their luggage through the Toronto airport—while Andrew walked down the corridor to meet his mom, Mary!

On the phone, Doug said, "We all cried like babies. Even airport security brushed back tears when they realized what was happening."

Since then, Andrew, who takes the medicine twice daily, has improved so much he rides a bicycle. If God intended kids to walk, he would not have allowed the invention of the bicycle.

Talking about God, what bothered me was Doug and Mary's attitude. Doug said, "It's a God-given miracle." Mary said, "My prayers have been answered. Doctor Patten got Andrew to walk."

In my view, God had very little to do with this cure. Denying me full credit troubles me and reveals a weakness in my character. What happened was not a miracle. It was another demonstration of the benefits of the direct application of science at the bedside and an excellent example of how covering all the bets, like finding the vitamin and iron deficiencies, in other words, managing the whole patient as a complex system and not just managing the muscle part, increases the probability of success. On the other hand, Mary and Doug believe it was their faith in God that led them to keep trying to help Andrew. So, by an indirect mechanism, you could argue faith did play a role in Andrew's recovery.

The newspapers reported what happened and so did CNN and TV. The article I like best is the one with pictures that appeared in the National Inquirer by James McCandlish (see documents). The papers reported Doctor Andrew Engel of the Mayo Clinic said he did not know why Doctor Patten was so much more effective than he was. Doug had an answer to that question: "Doctor Patten covered all the bets. He was not afraid of work and thinking. He was easy to talk to, kind, understanding, very thorough, and a good listener. He connected with Andrew on my son's level and with us on ours."

Whew! When I read that, tears came to my eyes. It was the best summary of the attributes patients need from a physician. In the future I shall try to measure up to that high standard. What I liked best was Doug had told the reporters I had treated them as a friend and not as a stranger.

But I didn't like how the media handled the recovery. The press made it look like a miracle. Instead, they should have informed the public that Andrew had a defect in neuromuscular transmission—a defect specifically corrected by ephedrine. In addition, because of difficulty swallowing, he was deficient in multiple vitamins and in iron. No magic was involved, and this was not a miracle. "There are no miracles," said Saint Augustine.

Fall Out

There was fall out. Some Nazi nurse reported me for doing magic tricks on rounds. Doctor Stanley Appel, the department chair, appointed a committee of five neurologists to investigate this behavior.

Me: "I do magic tricks for the kids and for the elderly. The purpose of the tricks is to neutralize the high-tech environment of the hospital and to show my human face. Besides, it's fun. 300 years ago, the great British physician Thomas Sydenham said, 'the arrival of a clown exercises more beneficial influence upon the health of a town than 20 asses laden with drugs.' An experienced physician knows the domain of science extends only so far. The majority of patients need the human touch. Andrew needed magic tricks, and that's what he got. So what!"

All neurologists on the committee voted to issue the following statement: "Nothing Doctor Patten did on rounds is incompatible with his personality."

A true statement! I took it as an endorsement.

Jim Killian, now vice chairman, said, "Now I suppose you will be doing magic tricks and juggling on rounds."

Me: "Not a bad idea, Jim. I'll have to take juggling lessons."

Stan, the chairman: "There will be no more investigations of your behavior." He added the national and international publicity about Andrew's recovery was "good." And that was that.

Lesson: There is a place in medicine for magic tricks. Bring in the clowns.

Experience with Myasthenia Gravis Goes Back to High School

Let's get back to myasthenia gravis, the topic before the digression about the investigation for doing magic tricks on rounds.

My experience with myasthenia went way back to high school because I knew a girl who had the disease. We didn't talk about myasthenia then. Such things were not discussed in polite company or at the dinner table. Her name was not Alice, but that is what I will call her because her family might not like my telling her story.

Alice Lief

She was cow heavy and fat, and she was ugly too, with one droopy eyelid and a sagging face and puffy everted lips. When she looked at you, her left eye stared straight out, but her right eye was cocked to the right, so she looked like she was looking forward and to the side at the same time. This gave her the hideous appearance of a medieval gargoyle, like the ones you see on the façades of ancient cathedrals, designed to scare off evil spirits.

In 1957, because of crowding with baby boomers, Van Buren High School in Queens Village, New York, had to go on triple sessions. With the other members of the track team, I got the early session, starting at 6:30 AM and ending at noon, so we could spend the afternoon at track practice.

Practice took place at Alley Pond Park along a five-mile course coach "Doc" Elstein and I had laid out the year before. The course was grueling, crisscrossing the terrain of the glacial moraine overlooking the vast Jamaica Plain. It was a great place to practice because it simulated Van Cortland Park in the Bronx, where the championship races took place. The disadvantage was it was miles from my home, so each afternoon I had to walk home exhausted with sore and trembling legs. Thank God, along the way, there was an oasis of refreshment, Lief's store and soda fountain. The store on the corner of Springfield Boulevard and 90th Avenue, next door to McHugh's Bar and Grill, was owned by Alice's mother and father. The store also carried other goods, groceries, and candy. Looking back on it, I now realize it was a kind of convenience store before the chains took over. Since the Liefs were the "other kind"—namely Jewish—and ours was an Irish Catholic neighborhood, most of our neighbors refused to buy there. But my mother, a maverick of sorts, didn't care. She claimed at Lief's there was an excellent rapport between price and quality, and she regularly made small purchases.

Lief's had a telephone booth, so I would go there when I wanted to talk with my girlfriends in private, without my mother and father listening. And together with the usual Happy Surprise and other candies, Lief's sold Duncan and Cheerio Yo-Yos, paddles with a rubber ball attached with a rubber string, and pink Spaldeens, our neighborhood's favorite ball for corner handball, street stickball, Ass ball, and front stoopball. I never bought cigarettes there except when mom wanted her Ivory Tipped Marlboros.

(Note: Ass ball is handball where the loser has to put his ass up and the winner gets to throw the Spaldeen at that ass. This game is called A-ball in the Bronx.)

At Lief's the usual thing was, when I arrived, hot and sweaty, a bell rang as I opened the door, and usually Alice came out from behind a dingy black curtain that separated the store proper from the back rooms where her family lived. I ordered my usual: a devil dog and an egg cream. I don't blame you if you don't know what they were because anyone who had not grown up in Queens would know nothing about them. The devil dog, the size of a hot dog, was two slices of devil's food cake with a whipped cream center, and the egg cream was a frosted glass of ice-cold water to which had been added just the right amount of vanilla syrup and a splash of milk. It cost six cents, the devil dog five, but that hardly mattered because in those days I was extraordinarily rich, clearing a weekly $3.10 profits from my Queens Village Review paper route. With tips, I often cleared over $5.00.

When I, cooling drink in hand, sat there in the shadowy dark interior of the soda fountain, firmly nested on a black vinyl stool, elbows perched on the cold black marble counter, black as onyx, reflecting on my silvered shadowy dark image in the frosted mirror across the way, I knew I was as close to the throne of heaven as I would ever come.

Alice never talked. One time, when I asked her how she learned to make such a wonderful egg cream, an enigmatic smile that tried to curl up the corners of her mouth involuntarily turned into a snarl, and she made a mumbled, low-pitched animal grunt, which had such pathetic overtones that I stared at her for a moment. Frightened, she ran back through the black curtain.

A few weeks later, I discovered what she had. I was watching Uncle Fred's cartoon show on channel 13 on our old nine-inch DuMont TV, when a public service announcement interrupted the program. There on the diminutive screen was a woman almost the spitting image of Alice, a woman with a droopy eyelid, skewed eyeballs, puffy lips, and a sagging face, who was saying in a muffled, low-pitched grunt, "I have myasthenia gravis." That afternoon I put a week's paper route profits in an envelope and sent it to the Myasthenia Foundation in Manhattan, the way the TV spot said I should.

My happy life continued this way for a few weeks more, with Alice acting as my personal servant and making the egg creams just right, and then, without warning, she disappeared.

Old Man Lief himself started making the egg creams. He was a short fat bald man with an obvious depression. His face was sad and had the dejected 'havior of the visage.' He didn't say much, but after four days he spoke and asked, "How do you like your egg cream?"

Without thinking, I said, "It's OK, but Alice makes it better." Lief hurled back. Shrieked. It was as if he were struck by a bolt of lightning. His face contorted and he let out a giant sob, and then he started crying uncontrollably. Lady Lief rushed out from behind the black curtain, hugged him, pressing her face close to his, and screamed at me. "What did you do? What did you do?"

"Nothing," I replied. "Just told the truth: Alice makes better egg creams. I didn't mean to offend him." Lady Lief came out from behind the counter and shook my hand and ushered me to the door.

"Where's Alice, anyway?" I demanded. "Why can't she make my egg creams?"

"Alice is sick. She is in the Mount Sinai Hospital in Manhattan. You did nothing. Don't worry about it."

"The myasthenia gravis is getting worse. I'm sorry," I said.

Lady Lief caught her breath and looked at me, amazed I could know about such a rare and unusual disease. She cleared her throat and choked. She was crying, I think. If she wasn't crying, she was about to because her eyes were wet. "You come here anytime you want. You're always welcome. From now on the egg creams and the devil dogs are free."

The next day Lady Lief made the egg cream and refused payment. "Alice's friends eat and drink here for free. Please tell the others," she said.

Three weeks later, Alice was back, but I could tell the myasthenia was getting worse. This time both eyelids were droopy, and the right almost covered her crooked eye entirely. She was having trouble keeping her head up and her breathing was rapid, shallow, and difficult. She almost couldn't lift the egg cream to the counter and with difficulty stirred the milk into the cooling drink. But she did stand there in the shadow behind the candy trays, looking at me with her straight eye, and I knew if her facial muscles had been strong enough, if she could have smiled, she would have been smiling then. I had my VB (VB = Van Buren High School) track letter sweater on, as usual, to impress the girls, and deep down in the core of my being, in the deep heart's core, I knew she was impressed. I knew Alice loved me—and in my own way, I believe, I loved her back.

Two days later there were no more egg creams for me. Lief's oasis of refreshment was closed. The next day there was a black crepe-paper wreath on the door.

At age 16, Alice Lief, the myasthenic and the best egg cream maker I ever knew, had died—died for all time.

Whew! Every time I think of Alice, I cry. That experience is the probable reason I did my medical school thesis on myasthenia gravis. The thesis was entitled Myasthenia Gravis: Possibly an Autoimmune Disease of Man. The thesis itself was full of circumstantial evidence, no real hard science. But it was right. Myasthenia gravis is now the best understood autoimmune disease of mankind. The treatments are directed against the autoimmunity and are often effective. One of those treatments was pioneered by one of my great mentors, W. King Engel at the Medical Neurology Branch of the National Institutes of Health.

Tableau Seven:

Medical Neurology at the National Institutes of Health and the Discovery of an Effective Treatment for Myasthenia Gravis

W. King Engel was the chief of the medical neurology, and I was his assistant chief. We were trying to discover treatments for myasthenia gravis, but it was a patient who made the discovery for us. She had myasthenia gravis, and she had been treated with prednisone for asthma. She claimed the myasthenia got much better during the treatment and worsened when the prednisone was stopped. "You doctors might try prednisone," says she.

King decided to try the prednisone on other myasthenia patients, and it worked on them too. In fact, it worked so well we did not need a double-blind controlled study or statistical analysis to demonstrate the beneficial effect. Our published papers on the subject and the awards won from the Myasthenia Gravis Foundation speak for themselves.

Neurologists Resist the New Treatment

What got me was the tremendous resistance of neurologists to use the new treatment. Here we had something that worked for a very serious disease, and yet the skeptics were unwilling to even try it on their patients. The major objection came from the myasthenia gravis center at the Mount Sinai Hospital in New York City. The myasthenia service there was, at the time, known worldwide for its excellence, and I had visited with Gabriel Genkins, the head doctor, several times to get pointers on how they handled their patients. All of a sudden, Gabe was against me and against King. To this day, I believe it was professional jealousy.

Lesson: Plato said the people who despise and defame shoe cobblers are the other cobblers. They do so out of jealousy and because the other cobblers are the competition. No one else besides the cobblers really cares or gives a damn. The delay in the general use of the new treatment for myasthenia was, in my opinion, the direct result of professional jealousy and an attempt by some physicians to keep patients for themselves. This, in my view, is a distinct failure and a violation of the Hippocratic Oath.

Truth wins out in the long run. Immune suppression in the form of prednisone and other agents is the worldwide treatment of choice for myasthenia gravis.

Talking about worldwide treatment reminds me of a famous myasthenic patient who died of the disease in Paris. The prednisone treatment didn't help him because he never got it.

Aristotle Socrates Onassis Dies of Myasthenia Gravis, and a Chauffeur Gets Kicked in the Pants in Portugal

Baylor College of Medicine

Harold Zierler, the director of the Myasthenia Gravis Foundation, had an idea. Harold's idea was based on our presentations and published papers that the prednisone treatment worked best in old men. So, Harold asked King if King would consider going to Paris to take care of Aristotle Socrates Onassis, who had myasthenia and was an old man. At the time, Onassis was in the intensive care unit of the American Hospital of Paris in Neuilly sur-Seine. You may have seen pictures of him with the tape he had applied to hold up his droopy eyelids. His tapes were white and stood out against his darker skin. Most patients used transparent tape so the tape would not be so obvious.

King didn't want to go to Paris, and I know why, and I don't blame him.

But I did. I love Paris in the springtime, etc.

"My bags are packed. Make the arrangements," I told Harold.

Harold was pretty sure the prednisone would pull Onassis out of a deep dark hole. Me too. I was sure I could cure Onassis. The apparent miracle would prompt the billionaire to express his gratitude by giving the Myasthenia Foundation and me and King money supporting myasthenia research. Without money these days, you can't do medical research. Without money, you can't wiggle.

So, Harold and I had a great strategy. But it didn't work! The best-laid plans, as the poet Robert Burns says, often go awry.

Harold tried to contact Onassis to get the big "OK." But they wouldn't put Harold through. Harold had to speak with Jackie. And that was that.

Harold and I were dumbfounded because Jackie said no and said no in no uncertain terms. She didn't want the new treatments, and she would sue us if we mentioned anything to her husband about them. Harold and I concluded Jackie wanted Aristotle dead. Whether that conclusion was justified or not, I don't know. The fact was Jackie vetoed our intervention, and by her command prevented her husband from receiving a free expert consultation and treatment. Yes, expert! By that time, we at the National Institutes of Health had more experience treating myasthenic patients with prednisone than any other physicians in the world. Experience is a great teacher, and I had the experience. Why not brag about it?

March 15, 1975, Onassis died at age 69. The cause of death is listed as respiratory failure as a complication of myasthenia gravis. That sounds fishy. No myasthenic should die of respiratory failure. If they can't breathe, put them on a respirator to breathe for them. Some countries do not have respirators, but that was not the case in France in 1975. Looking back on these events, the dark side of me wonders if money influenced Jackie's decision. Onassis gave Jackie $3 million to make up for the $3 million of the Kennedy trust she lost when she remarried. After Onassis' death, Jackie got $26 million and $150,000 each year for the rest of her life. The settlement was negotiated by Ted and grew under the stewardship of Jackie's companion, Maurice Tempelsman.

Visiting Professor in Lisbon, Portugal

Talk of respirators reminds me of the time (1970) when I was a visiting professor at the main Social Security Hospital in Lisbon, Portugal. We were making rounds with the hospital staff, including the director, and came across a myasthenia gravis patient who was having difficulty breathing when I suggested, "Just put her on a respirator." The director informed me, "There is no respirator in all of Portugal."

Later on, we discussed the treatment of a woman with puerperal sepsis, a common infection after childbirth and one often fatal if untreated. Most of the discussion, to my amazement, centered around the cost of treatment, which at the time amounted to about $27. Was she worth the cost? No kidding. This was a serious discussion because supplies of penicillin, and everything else, were limited. I volunteered to pay, but they would not have that. The director gave the orders to start the penicillin.

Rounds continued. I told the director I needed to stop into the patients' restroom to urinate. He said that restroom is way too dirty for me to use and referred me to the physician's bathroom.

Yee gods! The physician's bathroom was the dirtiest, filthiest, most mephitic smelling bathroom I had ever seen. There was shit on the walls and the floor and toilet paper and rotten food, oranges, lettuce, decaying cabbage, and other rubbish everywhere. If that was the doctors' bathroom, I can imagine what the patients' bathroom looked like. It had to be worse. Else why would they steer me away from the patients' bathroom to the doctors'?

The director announced the hospital had just gotten an electrocardiograph machine, but they did not know how to work it.

"Would you please show us how to hook up the electrocardiograph?"

"Of course, I will. I have had mountains of experience taking EKGs as an intern. I will have things up and running in a few minutes."

When they brought out the machine, my heart sank. The machine was one of those old Einthoven voltameters, a real antique in America—a museum piece, nothing less. I couldn't figure out how to hook it up or make it work, although I knew the principle involved the Einthoven triangle—electrodes had to be on both arms and at the pubis. The string didn't defect as it should with each electrical depolarization of the heart, and nothing showed on the rotating paper drum. I tried to explain my incompetence by telling them this was an old machine invented by Willem Einthoven, the Dutch physiologist who won the Nobel Prize for the invention.

"Ugh! I am so sorry. Such machines had been replaced and were no longer in use in the United States. Consequently, I have had no experience with them and don't know how to make them work. I'm not even sure this machine is actually working properly. The trouble could be with the machine or with me or with both the machine and me. Sorry!"

The hospital director said nothing. He just stared at me in disbelief and turned up his nose. Thus, rounds ended on a sour note. I could tell the medical staff was beginning to question how qualified I was to teach them anything.

Delicious Food and Wonderful Drinks

Lunchtime found us in the director's limousine headed into town to a famous restaurant, which I think was named The Frog, Il Frogua, something like that. Along the way, the limo stopped working, and the driver pulled over to the side of the road and opened the hood. Thus, we had another machine that wouldn't work. Then, the director started delivering well-directed strong kicks to his chauffeur's ass. Accompanying the kicks were shouts in Portuguese, which I gather were curse words.

Another limo arrived from somewhere and we went on to have the best luncheon I have ever had. During lunch, I sat next to a physician who had been an endocrine fellow at Harvard for two years. He asked me, "When I was in America, I saw Americans are always eating, and they are usually always eating shit. Why?" I replied, "I don't know. But you are right. Most Americans eat junk foods. This lunch is a thousand times better than any I have ever eaten in America. The roasted sardines are so good, and the Rosé wine is so delicious I will remember this great meal for the rest of my life."

And I have remembered.

Portugal is a different country. They do things differently there. Every country has its pluses and its minuses. In Portugal, lunch was a big plus, especially for me who embraces anything edible and anything alcoholic. Form your opinion of their country as you will. I have mine. And by the way, the Portuguese physicians have an opinion about the United States of America: "America is the best and the worst."

Lesson: Every country is different. Travel is a great eye-opener and will enlarge your experience of the world. Travel is transformative, and it's fun.

Lesson: On a recent visit to Portugal, I asked my brother Jim to suggest a good restaurant. His reply: "Any restaurant in Portugal." He was right. A trip to Portugal is highly recommended. The food is great, the wines are great, the people are nice and there is lot to learn from the museums.

Tableau Nine:

The Belgian Family Who Suffered Because They Misunderstood French in French Polynesia

Baylor College of Medicine
The Rich Belgian Family and the Dutch Crew

In 1988, the Alley Theater in Houston had a silent auction where you place bids on different things, and if you were the highest bidder, you got that thing. Ethel and I placed a small bid (I think $800) on a week-long vacation in Rangiroa, all expenses paid. Neither she nor I knew where Rangiroa was, and this was the first time we had become aware of the existence of the place. It turns out it is an atoll, the second largest in the world, and is located in the Tuamotu Archipelago, French Polynesia in the southern Pacific Ocean, 220 nautical miles north-northeast of Tahiti. In the Tuamotuan language, Rangiroa means "big sky."

Bingo! We were the highest bidders on that item and thus entitled to a vacation for a week in the South Pacific, all expenses paid. We were also the lowest bidders on the item because we were the only bidders. Probably people didn't know where or what Rangiroa was about, so they didn't want to bid. Too bad for them and very good for us.

A wonderful vacation in French Polynesia—ah, that was the theory. In practice, the travel agency that had sponsored the bidding reneged. They advised us to just chalk it up to experience and take the $800 which we paid to the Alley off our income tax as a donation to charity. They told us it would be way too much trouble and way too expensive for them to arrange such a vacation.

Ugh! There is way too much bullshit and financial fraud out there for us to lend any support to that sort of thing, and besides, we wanted our vacation for our 25th wedding anniversary, which would come in 1989.

Frankly, the Alley Theater and the travel agency were responsible for the item as advertised and either they performed, or the law would make them perform. Refund of money was out of the question because French Polynesia is very expensive and the vacation planned would have cost $638 per day at the one hotel on Rangiroa (Kia Ora), and there was a matter of airfare to Tahiti on UTA (an 18-hour ride) and airfare from Tahiti to Rangiroa and return. Thus, I estimated the true cost of the vacation would be $638 x 7 = $4,466, plus $1,800 airfares, plus our meals. The Alley and the Travel Agent had gotten themselves in a pickle, and they were not getting out.

It was one of the best vacations we have ever had. They have a lagoon there that is world famous, and a major motion picture was made in the lagoon, The Blue Lagoon. They also have a unique experience for the brave tourist. They drop the tourist into the water at the entrance to the atoll just at the moment when the tide comes rushing in. At that moment, the water moves at more than 70 miles an hour, and you are pushed ahead with tremendous force. The same force prevents the sharks from bending sideways to eat you, and you, thus, are swimming with the sharks, free of the fear of getting eaten. Once in the middle of the atoll, the Kanaka men fish you out of the water before the sharks get their bearings. Ethel took some wonderful pictures of me swimming among the sharks. Of course, I had plenty of experience swimming among the sharks at the Baylor College of Medicine.

Back to The Rich Belgian Family and the Dutch Crew

In the middle of our stay on Rangiroa atoll on a Wednesday, our hostess said, "They're really rich," focusing her eyes across the green lagoon to the bright white yacht moored there (see photo). "They come and go as they please and often sleep past noon."

Our hostess, the hotel manager, rolled her eyes and fixed her face in that kiss-pout, the French face of envy. "They really have the life of ease," she said, exhaling her harsh Gitane smoke into the soft Polynesian breeze.

The family came to dine with us. The trophy wife was young but bored. The man was gray and bent. Their little girl was happy for the change but had no friends.

They told me they and the crew were sick for a week and very weak, and their lips and tongue were numb. They were so weak they couldn't do a thing but sleep, and they often slept past noon. The captain came ashore to ask for help. The Kanakas and the Ray Rays (local natives are called Kanakas; Ray Rays are men raised and dressed as women, a Polynesian tradition going back for centuries) told him where to find me.

"You are a doctor! Please come visit us."

I did. And that was good luck for them.

Reader, did you figure it out? How did the crew and the passengers in a week's time get weak while cruising the South Pacific?

Answer: This rich family was Belgian, but their crew was Dutch. Their main problem was they didn't speak French well enough. They knew there was a poisonous fish in the area, a fish they were not supposed to eat. When they were told "Ne pas manger le puffer," they thought they heard, "Ne manger que le puffer." Don't eat the puffer versus only eat the puffer. Only eat the puffer would, of course, be poor advice and just the opposite of the intended warning about the poisonous pufferfish.

The Belgian Family Who Suffered Because They Misunderstood French

Since the only fish they ate for a week was puffer, they had developed serious puffer-fish poisoning. The tetrodotoxin toxin, stored in the fish liver and muscle, blocks the sodium channels in human muscle, making the victims weak. Severe pufferfish poisoning can be fatal due to respiratory arrest. Within a day of my treatment, the passengers and crew felt better. Complete recovery occurred soon thereafter as I thought it would and predicted. The family sponsored a gigantic banquet, not only for us but also for everybody at the hotel—tourists and hotel staff. The case was quite a coincidence because, I'll bet, though there were probably plenty of dermatologists around on vacation in the South Pacific, I was the only neurologist within 900 square miles.

Next question: what was my treatment that cured the passengers and crew of their weakness?

Answer: ne pas manger le puffer. Don't eat pufferfish. The passengers and crew recovered when they started eating a normal diet and stopped eating pufferfish. The beauty of this treatment is everything returns to normal when the cause of the weakness is removed. Of course, there are a variety of drugs and medicines that would have helped reverse the weakness induced by the pufferfish toxin, but why bother? One of my favorite treatments is to keep my hands in my pocket and do nothing. Most illnesses recover by themselves, so Rx nothing is usually not a bad idea, and Rx nothing usually has no side effects.

The Pufferfish Toxin is Insensitive to Heat

Tetrodotoxin is a heat-stable toxin, so cooking does not destroy its power. It is present in pufferfish (fugu), newts, goby, and frogs. As stated, it blocks action potentials in excitable cells by interfering with the increase in sodium permeability associated with excitation without any effect on potassium permeability. Human paralytic disease follows ingestion of toxic fish, but the bite of the blue-ringed octopus (also known as the blue-lipped octopus), whose salivary glands contain maculotoxin, a substance with an effect identical to tetrodotoxin, has also caused human deaths. In fact, the newspaper, Tahiti Pacifique, had a report of an American marine on R&R who found a small octopus in the blue lagoon and placed the octopus in his swim trunks so he would have his hands free. While walking on the beach, the marine let out a screech and told his friend, "the damn thing bit me." Those were his last words before he keeled over dead. That octopus had to have been the blue-lipped type. The marine learned the hard way the octopus's bite is deadly.

> **Lesson:** If you happen to meet up with a blue-lipped octopus, have nothing to do with it unless you're intent on suicide.

In Japan, there are special restaurants licensed to prepare fugu and special chefs who train for years and take written and oral tests to prove they can prepare puffer-fish safely. The Japanese men like the feeling of not being fully able to control their limbs when the fugu has taken hold. The effect, they say, is like being drunk but the thinking is not affected. Each year, there are a few deaths from fugu. Some are suicides and others from accidental ingestion of puffer liver, which concentrates the toxin.

While we are on this topic, try your skill on the next patient. See if you can get the diagnosis and prescribe a good treatment.

Baylor College of Medicine
Another Myasthenic Syndrome

You are called to see a 67-year-old man in consultation. He was in the recovery room after a prostate operation and seemed to be doing fine. He told the nurses he felt fine and asked for a glass of water, which he drank without difficulty. About 30 minutes after receiving an intramuscular injection of the antibiotic colistin, he became unable to move his arms and legs and then developed the inability to chew, swallow, talk, and breathe. His pupils dilated and did not respond to light. He was placed on a respirator and is conscious because he is able to answer simple questions by slight nods of his head.

Your diagnosis, please.

Antibiotic-Induced Muscle Weakness

Among the many side effects of antibiotic treatment is antibiotic-induced myasthenia, which occurs with neomycin, streptomycin, kanamycin, polymycin, bacitracin, dihydrostreptomycin, colistin (the culprit here), tobramycin, and amikacin. Each can produce paralysis, as was the case in this patient. Usually, the patient is an old man who has had some kind of urinary tract disease. They are the ones who get antibiotics right after operation to prevent infections. The disorder differs from natural myasthenia in that the pupils dilate, and the bladder loses its tone. Pupils and bladder are normal in natural myasthenia gravis.

How about treatment? Any ideas?

There is no good treatment to reverse the antibiotic-induced weakness, and such patients need support, particularly respiratory support, until the antibiotic has been metabolized. My job was to reassure the patient he would soon recover and to reassure the surgeon who was also frightened his patient had become quadriplegic. The treatment is to keep my hands in my pockets and to stop the colistin.

Result

The colistin was stopped and the patient supported. The paralysis lasted two days, and the patient thereafter thought he had pretty much returned to normal muscle function. Vancomycin, which has no neuromuscular blocking effect, was given after his muscles recovered. The paralysis did not recur.

Tableau Ten:

The Engineer Who Didn't Want to Pay His Bill

Baylor College of Medicine
Engineer X

It was a typical Thursday afternoon with a clinic packed with patients when I got a phone call in the exam room. The rule is no calls unless from a doctor. But it wasn't a doctor on the other end. It was a woman, a worried wife.

She: "Doctor Patten, please see my husband today. He is very sick, and I feel if you don't see him today, he will die."

Me: "How the devil did you get this number?"

She: "I don't know. I just dialed hoping you would answer, and you did."

Me: "Clinic is full. Most of these people have waited three months or more for their appointment. Talk with Cora and get on the schedule." (Cora Clay was my secretary, and, in my opinion, the best secretary in the world. Cora must have given this woman the number. Cora has extremely good judgment. So, I had better listen up.)

She: "I am so sorry to bother you. I know that will be too late."

At that point, tears came to my eyes, and a strange chilly feeling moved down my spine. There was an ache in the pit of my stomach. This poor woman needed me and needed me in a desperate way. "Bring him. I will see him right away." She was so nice. I am a sucker for a woman crying. Like Pop (my father), I was and am a sucker for a sob story. It might be a genetic Irish thing. I consider it a defect.

The nurses were put on the alert, and they put the patient (the woman's husband) in an examining room as soon as he arrived. It turned out I was the fourth neurologist the couple had consulted in the last two weeks. Each time, the wife was told her husband was psychologically ill and pretending he was physically sick when he wasn't. The wife gave it for her opinion the skiing accident her husband had had six weeks ago was doing something to his brain.

Me: "Skiing accident?"

She: "He took a hard fall on his butt. But after the fall, he was complaining his head hurt much more than his butt. Two weeks later, he seemed to be a different person. I don't know how to tell you he was different, but I have lived with him for 35 years, and I know he is—not himself."

> **Lesson:** Listen to the wife. She is telling you the diagnosis.

Whew! No better example of the benefit of and importance of getting a history. My routine physical exam and neurological exam was skipped. Instead, I had the patient walk for me. His gait was unsteady and on a narrow base. That was the reason the other neurologists thought he was hysterical. Organically ill patients usually walk on a wide base to steady themselves. Psychologically ill patients usually walk on a narrow base to make themselves look bad. So, this patient's gait looked hysterical, as if he had some kind of conversion reaction.

Notice I said organically ill patients usually walk on a wide-based gait. "Usually do" means "sometimes don't." He could be a patient with an organic illness who had not read the textbooks and consequently didn't know he was supposed to walk on a wide base and not walk on a narrow base. The complexity and variety of human experience are amazing. No two patients are alike, even if they have the same disease. In decades of medical practice, I have yet to see a typical "textbook" case of anything.

> **Lesson:** Textbooks are usually right, except when they are not.

Next came the fundoscopic examination with the ophthalmoscope. The optic nerve was swollen, and there were multiple hemorrhages there. Bingo! This man had increased intracranial pressure. With the history of trauma meant he probably had a subdural hematoma, a collection of blood under the fibrous connective tissue covering the brain. Blood in the subdural space can cause problems. The blood breaks down into smaller and smaller molecules. The increase in smaller molecules then sucks in fluid from the environment, causing the subdural hematoma (the blood clot in the subdural space) to expand and compress and displace brain tissue. Downward pressure from the expanding subdural hematoma can rupture bridging veins and cause more bleeding. Thus starts a vicious cycle that causes more displacement of the brain. Too much displacement will cause the brain to press on the brainstem and cause death by stopping those important brainstem functions like breathing, heart action, and blood pressure control.

His wife was right! This was an emergency. The most common emergency in neurosurgery. Her husband was about to die from an expanding subdural hematoma.

The Engineer Who Didn't Want to Pay His Bill

Lesson: Usually, the wife knows more about her husband's health than he does. It pays to listen to her. In no uncertain terms, the wife will tell you what is wrong.

"Cora, page Ed Murphy (the neurosurgeon). Put him right through to clinic."

Me: "Ed, drop everything. Tell them to clear out the CAT scan room. I am wheeling a patient over there for an emergency CAT. He has a subdural about to herniate."

This was many years ago when hospitals were different places. All I had to do was make a call, and everybody snapped to. There were no managers whose permission had to be sought. No insurance calls were needed to verify coverage or approve the scan. We just went to work doing our job.

Ed dropped everything and met me and the patient at the scanner. He, the radiologist, and I then saw the most amazing thing. During the scan, the brain shifted and pushed from right to left and down through the foramen magnum, compressing the patient's brain stem. There was a 23-millimeter shift from right to left at the level of the third ventricle. Normal is no shift at all. The lateral ventricle on the right was collapsed and the mesencephalic precisterns were occluded. Both of the patient's pupils dilated and did not respond to light. And the patient did not respond to any external stimulus—pinching, yelling, and so forth. He was in coma and at death's door. Those "fixed and dilated pupils," the famous FDPs of emergency rooms when the patient arrives DOA, dead on arrival, did not have, in this context, the same chilling prognosis. Ed and I were on the scene prepared to reverse events. In less than a minute, we would recall this engineer to consciousness and to life! We would save his life! About that, Ed and I had no doubt.

Why was the patient in coma? The reticular activating system is in the brainstem. Its job is to keep the brain awake. It was now knocked out, and the patient was unconscious because his reticular activating system was no longer working. The Glasgow Coma Scale rating is 3, the lowest possible, meaning eye, voice, and motor responses are absent. Still, I was not worried. The situation was perfect to save a life.

Ed did his thing. He put a hole in the patient's skull over the right-sided subdural. The old blood, now a liquid, squirted out under tremendous pressure and not quite hit the ceiling. The blood, as we expected, was colored dark brown like used machine oil. Dark liquid blood like that is characteristic of a chronic subdural hematoma, indicating the skiing accident six weeks ago was the probable event that caused the initial bleeding.

Ed took the patient, who was now awake but groggy, to the operating room for more clean out. The prognosis for full recovery was excellent. This man's wife had saved his life! Neurology can be more exciting than an Alfred Hitchcock movie. But here there was no artifice, no camera shots planned to terrify. This neurology adventure was real! Ah, how I loved saving a life. There is nothing like it, nothing as exciting, not even sex.

Neurosurgery Also Has a Dark Side

Neurosurgery has its pluses, its upsides, and this was one. It also has its minuses, its downsides. One down occurred when I was a neurology resident assigned to work with J. Lawrence Pool, who was the chair of the neurosurgery department at Columbia. He had a national and international reputation because he had written the foremost textbook about aneurysms and arteriovenous malformations (AVM) of the brain. Consequently, he got referrals from all over the world. One patient, however, a young housewife, came from close by—Scarsdale, a sleepy little village in Westchester, New York. She had developed a seizure disorder, and the arteriogram showed a massive collection of abnormal blood vessels in the non-dominant right hemisphere of her brain. Pool opened her head and cut and cut and cut. The brain does not come with dotted lines saying, "Cut here." or "Don't cut here." and arteriovenous malformations (AVM) look pretty much like normal brain. After the operation, Pool drew a beautiful multicolored diagram of the AVM he had removed and a picture of the brain after the surgery. He was an outstanding artist, and the patient's chart showed outstanding pictures of an outstanding surgical result. His note told of how he precisely, like a good surgeon, had cut where he did in order to precisely remove the AVM.

Me: "Gee, Doctor Pool, the operation was cool. What do you say we repeat the arteriogram and show how effective the surgery was? The films will make a big splash at the next grand rounds."

Pool: "Good idea, Patten. Go ahead."

After the arteriogram, I ran up the stairs with the films to Pool's office.

Me: "Doctor Pool, the AVM is still there—exactly as it was. We must have removed normal brain and missed the lesion completely."

The Engineer Who Didn't Want to Pay His Bill

Pool looked at the films, shook his head, and drew hard on his pipe. This is the way things sometimes were in the old days before CAT scan. You opened the head and somehow got into the wrong area and removed something entirely normal. Now you just don't get those errors (I hope) because of the absolute certainty of the diagnostic work-up. But in those days, Doctor Pool and I were staring at a painful reminder of our human limits as physicians and surgeons.

Me: "Doctor Pool, what do we do now? Should I put her on the schedule for a redo?"

Pool looks at me with a frown.

Pool: "No, Patten, that might upset her. Just send her home."

Me: "Should I tell her the AVM is still there?"

Pool: "No, Patten, that might upset her."

Follow-Up on the Engineer Whose Life Ed and I Saved

Several days after our big save, the patient left the hospital. Six weeks later, he came to clinic for a check-up. Everything was normal. But the patient had a complaint: "Doctor, you had some nerve sending me a bill for $660. What the devil did you do to earn that kind of money?"

Me: "I worried. Your wife worried, also. She will explain what happened. You had a health adventure you don't remember because you were too sick."

At the urging of his wife, the patient shut up. He paid the bill, though to this day he is amnesic of all the events you just read about. No one can blame him for not wanting to pay. Why should he pay when as far as he knows nothing was done? There is an interesting relation between our sense of time and memory. For this engineer, the time of his illness did not exist because he didn't remember it.

Lesson: Wives and marriage are important.

It has been known for a long-time married people live longer. Their married life together provides social support, of course, and touch therapy and sex—all those things probably play an important role in promoting wellness. But the main health advantage probably derives from watching out for each other. This is especially true for men, as illustrated by two cases. Men have a tendency to ignore important danger signals and avoid visits to doctors. Some examples:

One of my friends (a physician who should have known better) lived alone. One day, he happened to mention to his office manager he had been having severe chest pains for the last two weeks. His mention was two weeks too late, for my friend, right after making his statement, keeled over dead. A massive inferior lateral myocardial infarction (medical lingo for heart attack) was the cause of death.

On the other hand, another man woke up with weird pains in the side of his chest, face, and neck. He told his wife he would wait to see the doctor about the pains whenever he could get an appointment, probably sometime next week. The wife called 911. The patient had a dissection of the ascending aorta, which would have ruptured had it not been repaired surgically right away. The patient's wife was the cause of her husband's survival. Anything less than what she did would have been too little too late and would have resulted in the death of her husband.

A rarer event is when the wife gets sick, and the husband springs to action.

A woman became silent and then developed a paralysis of the right side of her body. She was at a family dinner when this happened. Her husband rushed her to the hospital where her speech and arm and leg function returned to normal after surgery. Diagnosis: Dissection of the carotid artery producing hemiparesis (paralysis of one side of her body) and aphasia (inability to speak). If this event had occurred while she was alone, the outcome might have been different.

Talking about my engineer with the subdural and his discontent with my fee makes me want to tell you about the biggest fee I ever collected from a patient. Unlike the engineer, he was happy to pay.

Tableau Eleven:

The Man from Saudi Arabia Who Wanted to Know Why He Had a Stroke

Baylor College of Medicine

He: "Doctor, I have been to Mayo, and I have been to Harvard. They told me I had a stroke. I knew that already. They told me the stroke was due to high blood pressure. That cannot be right. I never had high blood pressure. My pressure was, and is, normal. They have to be wrong. So, I am here hoping for you to tell me why I had the stroke."

Me: "Good."

The general physical exam showed he was in good shape. His neurological exam showed findings of a mild stroke affecting his right side with some slight weakness of the right hand and arm and some slowing of the ability to move fingers fast on that side. There was no sensory abnormality. Therefore, he had a pure motor lesion, caused by damage in a pure motor part of the brain, the internal capsule on the left side. And in fact, the scan showed the damage in the exact place predicted by the clinical exam. In fact, the damage was in the area most commonly associated with high blood pressure, and that is why the physicians at Harvard and Mayo Clinic told him his stroke was due to high blood pressure. They told him that because it probably was the truth. But how can you explain a stroke caused by high blood pressure when the patient did not have high blood pressure?

Lesson: When in doubt, take a history.

As usual, the history gives more information about the illness than most other things. The history often provides an answer to even the most puzzling clinical problems. When in doubt, take a history. Houston Merritt, one of the most famous neurologists of all time, was fond of saying, "Listen to the patient. He is telling you the diagnosis."

Me: "Tell me the circumstances surrounding the stroke."

He: "What do you mean?"

Me: "What were you doing, and where were you, and why, when you felt the weakness develop in your right hand and arm?"

He: "My friend and I go to London once a month and drink and have fun. At the time of the stroke, I was drunk in a London taxicab getting a blow job from a London prostitute. At the moment I came, had an orgasm, the weakness came with it."

97

Me: "What about your friend?"

He: "It's a funny thing, Doctor. My friend was in the cab with me. He was getting a blow job from another prostitute, and he had a heart attack at the same time. We took him to the hospital. He stayed three weeks. He recovered, but he takes heart medicine."

Me: "The stroke was caused by the tremendous elevation of blood pressure during orgasm. The heavy drinking has an adverse effect on blood clotting by impairing the function of platelets, which are needed to clot the blood. So, two things caused the stroke: The sudden increase in blood pressure at the time of orgasm and a compromised clotting system due to the alcohol. The area of the brain involved has a small artery, the thalamoperforating artery. It has a weak wall and can break under high blood pressure. So, in a certain sense, the doctors at Mayo and Harvard were correct. Your stroke was due to high blood pressure. In your case, the high blood pressure was temporary and due to the blow job orgasm. The good news is that the bleeding, for the most part, displaced brain fiber tracts and caused little permanent damage. Thus, your prognosis for full recovery is good. But if you go to London and drink a lot and engage prostitutes, it is possible, under similar circumstances, you might have another stroke."

The patient's wife, who had been in the room all this time listening to all of this very frank discussion of drinking and blow jobs, jumped out of her seat and kissed and hugged me.

He: "Doctor, I have $8,000 in cash. Will that be enough to cover your fee?"

Me: "My fee is $12,000. You can pay the difference with your credit card."

He: "$12,000! No one ever charged me that much. You must be the best neurologist in America."

Me: "Thank you. I appreciate what you said. I will check you in six months. Make an appointment at the desk."

Follow up: he and his wife returned for routine checks. He stopped drinking, and he no longer engaged prostitutes. He had no further trouble with strokes or blood pressure. His wife treated me as if I walked on water and hugged and kissed me each time they came to clinic. It is unethical (according to some) to let the wife of a patient do such things, but I let her do it anyway. The big fee was part of his treatment.

The Man from Saudi Arabia Who Wanted to Know Why He Had a Stroke

It was good for him to pay a big fee so he would follow and value my advice. The big fee was also good for me.

> **Lesson:** Listen to the patient. He is telling you the diagnosis.

Ethel (my wife) is an internist. She is fond of saying, "If all else fails, take a history." A good history often gives a clear picture of the patient and the problem. How in the world would we have known about the blow job stroke unless the patient told us? The trouble is history takes time, and time is money. So, some physicians cheat the patients on time to get more money on volume. That regrettable practice often starts a fruitless pursuit of irrelevant matters with a pile of tests. A good history will make more diagnoses than a hospital full of tests and many more miracles than a church full of saints. Most illnesses are not catastrophic. Time will provide the powerful answer of whether a condition needs further investigation. Years of experience taught me to keep my hands in my pockets and watch the problems solve themselves without further tests.

During the history, I like to have the wife in the room. The wife is important in focusing on the essential issues and conveying more truthfully what has transpired. I say wife rather than husband because women are more generally knowledgeable and informative about their husband's health than vice-versa. Several illustrations will follow.

According to the great clinician and medical researcher Bernard Lown, history is the most important aspect of doctoring. No time is spent more productively, and history is the foundation for a human relationship between patient and doctor based on mutual respect. The time invested in history is but a small sacrifice for curing and healing.

> **Lesson:** London must have some amazing prostitutes.

Sidebar about Saudi Arabia

I used to consult for ARAMCO. John, an American, who worked there had a rare muscle disease called dermatomyositis.

Neurology Rounds with the Maverick

Baylor College of Medicine
John of ARAMCO

John's dermatomyositis condition came under control with the usual treatments. One night at a party he, and his wife got into a tremendous argument. She took off in the family car, and he borrowed his friend's truck to catch up with her. Two miles down the road, the Saudi cops had already stopped the wife. Women were not allowed to drive in Saudi. My patient stopped to try to get his wife off the hook but ended up getting searched himself. The cops also searched his friend's truck. There they found a quart of whiskey, which in Saudi is like finding a kilogram of heroin in the United States.

John was arrested and spent the next three months in a Saudi prison. You can bet the prison was dark and dirty and stunk, and the food was lousy, and there were rats around, and so forth. It was a real purgatory, if not hell itself.

At the end of three months, a well-dressed man came to see John. He showed John a picture and said, "When you get to open court, point to the man in the room whose picture this is. Then say, 'That's him. He sold me the whiskey.' If you do that simple thing, you will be on an airplane back to the U.S. in the afternoon. If you don't do that, you will spend the rest of your life here in this prison."

"For God's sake. I told the other prosecutor. The truck wasn't mine. The whiskey wasn't mine. I don't know where the whiskey came from. I don't have any idea who sold it, and I don't know who bought it."

The well-dressed man just smiled. "You have a choice. Tell the story your way, and you end up staying here forever. Point to this man (he holds up the photo again), and you end up on a plane headed home."

The next day they took John to a courtroom. Suddenly the lights in the court dazzled his eyes accustomed to the dim dark prison cell. He looked around like an owl half blinded by bright daylight. John was still not seeing clearly when someone asked, "Do you see in this courtroom the person who sold you the whiskey?"

John looked around. Sure enough, the man in the photo was there in the prisoner's dock.

Ugh! What would you do, dear reader? Would you rat? Or would you not rat? To rat or not to rat—that is the question. More to the point: thou shall not bear false witness. That false witness commandment is clear and important. Bearing false witness has caused gigantic problems in our society. Fox News, for instance, in my opinion, is almost all false witness and false information, and misinformation riles up people who can't think for themselves. For about 50 years, the tobacco companies as a false witness told the public that smoking does not cause cancer or that there is no scientific evidence that smoking causes cancer or that there is no expert consensus that smoking causes cancer when it does, and they knew it did, and that the scientific evidence was overwhelming, and consensus was a fact. Jeffrey Wigand in 1996 went on 60 Minutes and disclosed that Brown & Williamson Tobacco Corporation had misled the public for years about the addictive and carcinogenic properties of cigarettes.

Vested economic interests lied to us about acid rain, DDT toxicity, lead in gasoline damaging infant brains, secondhand smoke causing asthma, the ozone hole caused by chlorinated fluorinated carbons, aspirin as a cause of Reyes disease, birth control pills and stroke, the local and systemic complications of breast implants, and, more recently, global warming.

Should John join the crowd and bear false witness? If he does bear false witness, this innocent man in prisoner's dock will suffer greatly.

What would you do, reader? Think!

I pause for reply.

John is now in my clinic office. He stares at me and asks, "What would you do, Doctor Patten?"

Me: "I don't know. Far be it for me to judge anyone. Everything is wrong from the start. The whole situation—it stinks. The women can't drive thing stinks, the whiskey is illegal thing stinks, the false arrest thing stinks, and trial of the man in the photo stinks. It all stinks to high heaven. It stinks that Saudi Arabia, a kingdom not a democracy, is supported by the United States government. I don't know what I would do. I don't. But I know what you did because, John, you're here."

John says nothing. He bows his head and then blots tears with a white tissue I have handed to him.

Tableau Twelve:
Eulogy to Bill

Baylor College of Medicine

Bill was referred by the ALS Society of America in California for diagnosis and treatment of what was thought to be ALS. ALS is amyotrophic lateral sclerosis, a fatal nervous system disease.

It was clear from the history and neurological examination Bill did not have ALS. He had a severe vasculitis, an inflammation of many blood vessels, including the blood vessels of the brain. The diagnosis was proven by arteriogram and biopsy.

This condition was suspected in clinic when I put my otoscope up his nose and saw the light put into one nostril came out the other nostril. Bill had a hole in his nasal septum, the tissue separating one nostril from the other. In fact, I could see the hole with my scope. It was the size of a dime and there was bleeding at the edges.

People who use lots of cocaine have problems with their noses for many reasons. The cocaine can constrict blood vessels and damage tissue that way, and some coke has small sharp crystals that can cut into tissue and do damage. When Stephen King talked about his cocaine problem in his book *On Writing*, he mentioned he had to plug both nostrils with tissue because of the bleeding. Whatever the exact mechanism of the nose hole and the bleeding, it was clear Bill was using cocaine and lots of it. Robin Williams famously said, "Cocaine was God's way of telling you that you are making too much money." Bill fit in with that idea because his media business was making oodles of money.

Because his type of vasculitis was known to be associated with cocaine use, the most probable diagnosis was cocaine-induced vasculitis. The treatment would have required Bill stop the stuff. If the vasculitis continued after the cocaine was stopped, then he would need some medicines to suppress the inflammation of the blood vessels.

But Bill had a different idea. He wanted to continue the coke. He said he wanted to commit suicide, but he was too chicken to hang himself or take an overdose of sleeping pills. He wanted to die the easy way by taking too much coke.

Me: "Why do you want to kill yourself?"

Bill: "This is a way of getting back at my father who has dominated and controlled my life up to now. This will be the final way I take control."

Result

Bill continued his downward course of using coke and died of his disease. Along the way, he went through a fortune, ruined his media business, and hurt his wife and family. Bill's death might have had an adverse effect on Bill's father, who was a giant in the TV business. Then again, it might not have had any effect at all. Who knows? Because I felt helpless in trying to help Bill, I wrote a poem about his situation. My medical care, in this case, was completely ineffective.

Eulogy to Bill Before His Big Scene

You hoovered your lines real well and convincingly evoked that ancient Bolivian God

Who explodes inside your head and then proceeds to eat your flesh, drink your blood, devour your media business, wife, and life to leave you dead.

As your physician, I observe with interest some signs of your addiction:

The scared, malnourished Asian stare,

The bloody nose hole black,

Door to the darkened universe,

These things are real; your story is the fiction.

Your stage presence falters as you explain with grim, grin, grimace,

The reasons for your acts.

By killing yourself, you are resolving your Oedipal complex the easy way.

"Things go better with coke," you say.

Once again, you fail to face the facts.

Rock and flake pound your brain

Reducing it to a critical mess.

Eulogy to Bill

Poem notes: Hoovered is the term used by cocaine addicts for the act of snorting the coke. It relates to a brand name vacuum cleaner and also reminds us of an American president who was overly optimistic when the U.S. was entering a great depression. The lines are both the lines in a play an actor might say and also the lines of coke as they are assembled on a surface before inhalation.

The bloody nose hole is part of the pathology induced by the cocaine in the nose, with perforation of the nasal septum. Black door to the darkened universe refers to a black hole where gravitation is strong and also sounds like "back door." A natural death would be a normal entrance to the world of the dead; a drug-induced suicide would be a back-door entrance.

"Rock" is the term for the free amine form of cocaine (crack), and flake is the most commonly available form. The poem, as mentioned, has references to Bill, who owned a now-defunct PR media firm and acted in his own commercials.

The English version of the poem and the French version and my picture were published in *The Trimestrial Poetry Review*, the official poetry journal of the European Union, July–August 1989, with some of my other poems in English and in French, pages 75–83. In the same journal appeared poems by Iosif Brodsky, Václav Havel, and Paul Celan. I am not in the same league as those poets, but my poems are in the same poetry journal.

Tableau Thirteen:

Patients Who Were Not My Patients but Still Interesting

Baylor College of Medicine
Ben Taub General Hospital

Ben Taub General Hospital is the Harris County Charity hospital where I used to supervise the neurology service on a part-time basis. What a collection of patients were there, and what unusual conditions!

Case One

Medical student William Copland and I were called to the emergency room to consult on a big-as-a-house black mama who was having back pain. The pain was severe and came in periodic intervals of eight minutes.

My sense of smell is excellent, and I smelled she was pregnant. The smell of pregnancy is a peculiar sweetish scent difficult to describe. In clinic, on multiple occasions, I smelled pregnancy and asked, "How long?" Sometimes the woman didn't even know she was pregnant. Always the tests agreed with my diagnosis made by smell. My daughter Allegra, who is also a neurologist, has the same ability to diagnose pregnancy by smell. I was going to publish a paper on this special diagnostic ability but decided against it because no one, except Allegra, would believe it.

Back to back pain in mama.

The lateral abdominal film showed the fetus had descended, and, in fact, MAMA WAS IN LABOR, hence the pain and hence the pain coming in periodic intervals.

"Bill, go over there and find out how she got pregnant," said I.

"Excuse me, ma'am, but Doctor Patten over there is the chief of the neurology service, and he wants to know how you got pregnant."

"It sure as hell weren't any skinny-dicked white boy like you!" came the reply. Mama had a sense of humor alright, and Bill Copland, who was on the small side, may have had a small you-know-what. Nope—change that. Bill probably did have a small you-know-what.

Further clarification from mama: "Two men lifted me up onto the kitchen table, and while they held me there and spread my legs, the third did the nasty."

Bill Copland went on to become a famous neurologist. You can ask Professor Google about him if you wish. When he asked me to write a letter of recommendation for him, I said in my letter, "Bill is the only person I know who can sing Yellow Submarine in Latin." This was, of course, a true statement. Bill and I used to trade turns reciting Virgil's Aeneid. He is the only medical student I have ever met who was fluent in Latin. He even could do book six. Bill Copland's website mentions, under the heading "Languages Spoken in Clinic," that he partly understands French but has a professional command of Latin. In fact, I am sure an ancient Roman patient, a Civis Romanus, would have no trouble talking to Bill.

Anyway, every interview for residency started right off the bat with a request for Bill to sing *Yellow Submarine* in Latin. That rendition was quickly followed by the offer of a residency position. How come? Who knows? My take is most program directors in neurology are bored stiff with their job and are burned out. Anything unusual and different is their cup of tea and most welcome.

Me too. My official Texas Physician website mentions I speak some Mandarin, serviceable French and Spanish, but fluent Latin. In the decades of practice, no Civis Romanus (cf. Cicero's In Verrem) has shown up—yet. I still can hope, can't I?

Case Two

A young man, 22 years old, was admitted in coma. The story was he was found unconscious under a bridge. Physical exam and neurological exam revealed nothing except coma and a brown nose. Coma means there was no response to stimuli, even painful stimuli like pinches and stabs with a needle. The brown material caked over his nose was greasy and had a faintly sweet aroma. It was not shit as some had assumed.

The CAT scan showed a massive round swelling in the right hemisphere of the brain. The mass was displacing midline brain structures to the left. The radiologists thought it was a brain tumor, probably a low-grade astrocytoma. Neurosurgical consults advised immediate operation to relieve pressure and to biopsy the tumor for diagnosis. And that would have happened if the kid had been admitted to the neurosurgical service. But the kid had not been admitted to neurosurgery. He was on neurology, and, therefore, we neurologists controlled the case and dictated what would happen.

My feeling was we don't open someone's head without a very good reason, and in this kid, we just didn't have a clear indication of what was causing the swelling, and, therefore, the better part of valor was to keep our hands in our pockets and just offer supportive care. Rx: watch and wait and do nothing except supportive care.

Supportive care is turning of the body by the nurses to prevent bed sores, cleaning up after the kid defecates, managing nutrition and electrolytes, controlling infection with antibiotics, and so forth.

The coma continued for another six weeks. And the nurses continued to do their thing effectively and with good cheer. Jesus, if we didn't have nurses, we would be up the creek. What would we do without them? Nurses are among the unsung heroes of our civilization. Praise them.

A New Group of Medical Students Arrives

One day, I was standing at the side of the kid's bed, addressing a new group of medical students. "What we need here at Ben Taub is a neurological detective to go out there and find out the connection between the bridge, the coma, the brain swelling, simulating a brain tumor, and the brown nose. The key to this case is the brown nose."

As if on cue, the patient sat up. The kid looked at me with a wry smile and said, "I can tell you. That day instead of the usual one bag of shoe polish, I inhaled three bags full. My favorite flavor is brown."

Our patient enjoyed inhaling shoe polish. He would spray the polish into a bag and then inhale the contents. His favorite flavor was (what else?) brown. Hence, the brown nose.

Sure enough, Medline listed eight other cases of shoe-polish-induced brain swelling. All the cases recovered with rest, as did our patient. This kid was just part of America's love affair with drugs. His drug of choice happened to be shoe polish, and his favorite flavor was brown. Former hippies understand the scene. What's your bag?

And so, the kid with the brown nose left Ben Taub fully recovered with his CAT scan returned to normal. Most of his physicians thought he would soon be back in the brown, but I hope not as much.

Case Three

The resident presented a new patient who had both syphilis and AIDS. "He is not a homosexual," said the resident.

"How do you know?"

"His earring is on the wrong side. His is on the left. The homosexuals wear theirs on the right. Right is wrong."

"Any idea where he got the diseases?"

"I didn't ask."

"You might try next time learning something about your patients."

So, we marched over to the patient's bedside. "Excuse me, sir, I am Doctor Patten. The residents here have been telling me about your troubles. You have AIDS, and you have syphilis. We will take care of the syphilis and expect to cure it. And we will do our best to help you control the AIDS. But we have a question. Where did you get these diseases?"

"That's easy," says the patient. "For six years, I have been having unprotected anal sexual intercourse with my brother. He has AIDS and syphilis."

"One more question: we see you are wearing a ring in your left ear. How come?"

"I haven't come out of the closet yet."

Lesson: Homosexuality is a biological and genetic issue—one that should not cause anyone feelings of guilt.

Case Four

Ben Taub has a prison ward where criminals are looked after. Part of the job of attending neurologist at Ben Taub was to consult on the neurological problems of the patients there. The residents were not allowed to do that for some reason, probably because they were not board certified and therefore not considered qualified to testify as experts in court should the need arise.

Patient Jesus

Jesus was his name, and Jesus had been very naughty. He had held up a 7-11 convenience store. When the clerk refused to turn over the money, Jesus shot the clerk in the chest. Jesus then drove two blocks south only to discover he was low on gas.

Jesus stopped at a Shell station and started to fill his tank when the attendant came out to ask for payment. Jesus shot and killed him too. Those are the facts. Within a 10-minute period, Jesus had killed two people. At the request of his lawyer and at the order of the judge, Jesus was admitted to Ben Taub General Hospital for psychological and neurological examinations.

Jesus claimed that he did not remember the 7–11, nor did he remember killing the clerk, nor did he recall killing the station attendant. Jesus said that he had a seizure disorder that caused him to lose consciousness, and under the influence of the seizure, the aforementioned bad things may have happened.

General physical examination, neurological examination, and all the usual tests were normal. The electroencephalogram was done in the routine manner and that being normal, I got electroencephalograms under activation techniques. The activation techniques are designed to bring out abnormal electrical brain activity that might be missed on routine electroencephalogram. Result: Jesus had normal brainwaves under conditions of sleep deprivation, hyperventilation, metrazol activation, and photic stimulation. As part of the evaluation, I also ordered measurement of auditory, visual, and somatosensory evoked responses. Thus, we effectively measured Jesus's nervous system in detail. Again, nothing showed but normal results. Thus, by all clinical and laboratory criteria, Jesus had a normal nervous system.

Court Testimony against Jesus

My testimony was damaging in the extreme. I told the jury there was no seizure disorder that could explain this criminal behavior. I gave it for my opinion Jesus had a normal nervous system.

His lawyer: "Do you mean to say, Doctor Patten, that you can state with absolute certainty my client does not have a seizure disorder?"

Me: "Yes, sir, that is what I am saying."

His lawyer: "Are you calling my client a liar?"

Me: "Yes, sir. I am calling him a liar. He is lying. I am calling him a liar because he has lied."

His lawyer: "Then how do you account for his not remembering anything about what happened."

Me: "He made up the amnesia story and the seizure story to get out of the punishment that he knows is coming his way. He made the whole thing up to suit his own convenience. He wants to avoid the needle. In my opinion, he remembers every-thing and just made up the story about not remembering." Notice in court I repeat myself while looking directly at the jury. That is a technique to make my testimony more believable. Repetition is not proof of anything, but I do it anyway because it is effective.

The judge dismissed me after the District Attorney on redirect hammered home my message that Jesus knew what he was doing and did not have a seizure disorder and was conscious and not unconscious, but fully conscious when he killed the men.

As I waited for the elevator, two police escorted Jesus down the hall. Jesus was in irons with chains around his legs and both hands cuffed in front. With Jesus in a state of restriction and confinement, he didn't scare me much. But I did back away.

Jesus looked at me and smiled. "You're right, Doc. I made the whole thing up."

Some people, including murderers in court, have no feeling of guilt or remorse. And some have a sense of humor and an attitude.

The jury said, "Guilty as charged." Jesus got the death penalty, what Jesus probably deserved for killing two people in cold blood. The death penalty is certainly a pen-alty—pretty permanent too.

Case Five

The neurology service was asked to consult on a patient on the surgical service who suddenly became completely hemiplegic after one of the junior surgical residents installed a tracheostomy to help the patient's breathing.

Neurological resident: "He is a 52-year-old completely unable to move his left side or feel anything on that side. Face, arm, leg—all gone. But here's the killer: whoever put in the trach tied off the carotid artery on the right side causing the stroke. Ugh! I don't know what to do. Should I write our Dx (diagnosis) in the chart?"

Me: "What do you think?"

Neurology resident: "It's the truth, but they're going to hate it. Might bring a mal-practice case."

Me: "Mistakes are made every day. This is just one of the most egregious. They con-sulted us to find out why this man had a sudden stroke. So, we should tell them. Write it and let the chips fall where they may."

Patients Who Were Not My Patients but Still Interesting

Telephone call from Doctor Gordon (not his real name, but the senior surgeon supervising the Ben Taub surgical service at the time): "God damn you, Patten. Are you crazy? Putting that in the chart! We could get fucking sued. You must be a moron."

Me: "It's the truth, right. Your boy tied off the carotid and caused the stroke."

Doctor Gordon: "God damn stupid thing, no question. We took the god damn thing off, but the patient is still stroked out, and the vessel is clotted all the way into the cranium. Hopeless, really."

Me: "Sorry. Mistakes are made. If we don't recognize our mistakes, we might make them again. I'm sure your resident will be more careful next time around and not tie off a large pulsating artery in the neck that could be the carotid. Our experience, as neurologists, is that an open carotid is needed to keep the brain functioning."

Doctor Gordon: "You are a nut case! MED will hear of this!"

And that was that. I never heard any more either from Doctor Gordon or from MED (Michael DeBakey, president of the Baylor College of Medicine and my boss).

The patient died from the massive brain swelling that follows a massive brain infarction. The family did not sue. Whether the family was told the cause of the stroke or not, I don't know. But the way things usually work out at Ben Taub, the family would not have sued even if they were told. At Ben Taub, charity went both ways. The patients loved their doctors, and the doctors loved their patients. That is altogether fitting and proper and the way things were structured in the golden age of medicine.

One Last Thing about Ben Taub

We, the residents, medical students, and I, had just finished rounds and had returned to the office. The previous day, there had been a reunion of Interns at Cornell Medical College in New York City. At the cocktail party at Sotheby's, I discovered there was to be an auction of paintings the following day. One of the paintings to be sold was The Bathers by Renoir. The recommended bid was between $20 and $37 thousand. Boasting to my Ben Taub entourage, I said, "As I am not a cheapskate, I placed my bid at the 37 thousand dollars and therefore expect to own, by the end of today, a beautiful Renoir."

While the interns and residents and medical students looked on, I phoned Sotheby's. Ugh! They sold my painting to the Osaka Museum of Art for $8 million! The best-laid plans of mice and men, etc.

Ward Service at the Neurological Institute of New York

Talking about Ben Taub reminds me of the charity ward patients at Columbia-Presbyterian Hospital in New York City. Some were just as interesting and should have their stories told. Ward service in New York in my day was like at Ben Taub, only no adult supervision (most of the time and very little adult supervision some of the time).

At the Neurological Institute in New York City in the old days, the residents had their own service. It was called the Ward, and there were four divisions. A resident could, if he wished, admit a patient to his own service and take care of the patient as his own. We didn't collect a fee. The hospital did the collecting if there were any fee, and there usually wasn't, as these patients were the poor of the city. Whereas the patients at Ben Taub were cases to me because I was not their physician, but was an advisor to the residents who were actually in charge, at Columbia the patients were my patients and not cases. Attending neurologists did make teaching rounds on the wards once or twice a week. They were available for free consultation on any patient but did not see all the patients and did not have the final say-so on patient care. At Neurological Institute, in those days, the attending neurologist gave advice and nothing else.

Patient 1

He was an army sergeant who stood at attention as I entered the examining room, and he stood there at rigid attention and pointed the index finger of his right hand at me as he told his story:

"You are the fourth neurologist I have consulted. None of the others helped. This is the last time I am going to tell my story. If you can't help me, I am going to kill myself. Understand?"

I nodded.

"Are you listening? I am going to tell this once, and only once. So, listen up."

I nodded again and sat down at my desk, folded my arms across my chest in protective gesture, and focused my attention on the patient. He was about six feet tall, in his thirties, had gray hair—completely gray hair, blue eyes, and a shield-like chest.

"Six months ago, I got tingling in my toes. The tingling spread to my fingers, to my wrists, and then marched up my legs to my waist. Then my pecker stopped working. After that, my legs got stiff, and I lost my sense of balance. In the dark, I must hold onto something or I will fall."

"May I ask a question?"

"Of course!"

"Has there been any fluctuation in your symptoms, or has it been a steady downhill?"

"Downhill every god damn day."

"Any trouble thinking?"

"No. Except I keep thinking someone might be poisoning me and that is why I am sick. Do you think someone might be poisoning me, or am I going crazy?"

"Unlikely. Both are unlikely. From the way you look and the story you told me, I think I know what's wrong and what to do about it. Let me examine you. Take off your clothes except for underwear. Put on this gown with the open end in back. I'll return in four minutes."

The examination showed all the expected features of his disease: loss of position and vibration sense in the lower extremities, poor balance, hyperactive reflexes, glove and stocking sensory loss, and so forth. All the features of combined systems disease, the neurological complication of pernicious anemia, a fatal disease if left untreated. The usual patient has no gastric acid and cannot absorb vitamin B12 from food. There are many causes of this inability to absorb B12, and it might be nice to find out exactly what the problem was in his case. So, I admitted him to the hospital for diagnosis and treatment.

Before clinic was over, the head nurse on Neuro 2 West called to tell me my new patient had arrived and had been admitted, all the paperwork was done, and he was now trying to sign out against medical advice. "He says we are trying to kill him, and he has to leave. Next time, Doctor Patten, will you please send these paranoid nut cases to psychiatry where they belong."

"Put him on."

"Doctor Patten, the nurses are trying to kill me, so I got to leave."

"Don't be silly. They are trying to help you, and so am I. The feeling you have is called paranoia. It is a mental problem. It goes with your disease. Stay there, and I will come talk with you as soon as I finish clinic. There are only six patients to go, so I can be with you in about an hour."

Ward Service at the Neurological Institute of New York

Before I got there, he left.

The next day he called and wanted to be readmitted, and he was. Only this time, he thought the dietician was out to kill him by planning to put poison in his food. Again, he signed out. Two more times he came and went, each time afraid someone wanted to kill him. He freaked out when the EKG (electrocardiogram) technician put on the electrode leads. He thought the test was a prelude to electrocution. He was under a delusion, a false belief not amenable to logical persuasion. Delusion, in this case, took the form of a paranoid idea hospital people were out to kill him. Actually, I thought he was afraid to die. He was afraid to die because he knew that his down-hill course was headed that way—to death. To compensate for this fear of death, he developed the mental mechanism of telling himself since the people in the hospital were trying to kill him, he could escape death by leaving the hospital. The reason that idea sounds crazy is that it is crazy—very crazy. It is crazy because it does not match up with reality. The trouble with crazy ideas like that is they don't work.

Crazy patients are never all crazy. There is always some element of sanity in them. The trick is to get that element to control the behavior. I can't recall how I persuaded him to stay, but I do recall his wild look, the haunting unpleasant look of panic. He believed people were out to kill him. Imagine how frightening it must be to think people are out to kill you.

Our United States Army sergeant agreed to enter the hospital, obey orders, and stay five days without mentioning his delusion and without trying to escape.

His hematocrit was 36%, which was normal for a menstruating woman from Spanish Harlem or someone with parasitos, but not normal for a red-blooded member of the United States Army. The expected hematocrit for a man was about 48–56%. And yet, the hematology consultant didn't want to do a bone marrow examination because he felt the 36% was normal. My argument that my hematocrit was 48% did not persuade.

Oh well, there were giants in the earth in those days, doctors who weren't afraid of their shadows or malpractice suits. Doctors who had guts. If the hematology resident wouldn't do the bone marrow, if he said it was not indicated and wrote that in the chart, so what! I knew someone who would do the bone marrow, someone I trusted, and someone my patient trusted. Namely: me!

The bone marrow was abnormal and proved the patient had the characteristic findings of pernicious anemia: megaloblasts filled the marrow, giant immature red blood cells, who weren't able to grow up to be normal red blood cells because they were deficient in vitamin B12.

Next came some tests to find out why my patient was deficient in B12. These were necessary, in my view, to better treat the condition. Some B12 deficiencies are due to serious diseases of the gut like lymphoma or amyloidosis or bacterial overgrowth in the gut causing poor absorption and so forth. To pinpoint the defect, the patient was given a capsule of vitamin B12 that had a radioactive cobalt at the center of the molecule. Cobalt is the metal at the center of every molecule of B12. In fact, the original form of the vitamin was probably a form of cobalt, and then, as evolution marched on, the other parts of the molecule were attached to help the cobalt do the job of transferring methyl groups and electrons and doing important whatnot in human metabolism.

The test showed no radioactive B12 in the patient's urine, indicating no absorption of B12. A repeat test with intrinsic factor (the stomach factor missing in patients with pernicious anemia) corrected the defect and restored B12 absorption to normal. Bingo—that was the diagnosis. The patient had B12 deficiency because he couldn't absorb B12 from food. He could not absorb the vitamin because his stomach was not making the stomach factor needed to absorb B12.

He: "I don't know what was in that last test, Doc, but that's the treatment I need."

It is such a wonderful feeling to know what is going on with a patient. The best prognostic factor is when the doctor knows what is happening. The worst prognostic factor is confusion in the mind of the physician. The treatment was to supply B12 by intramuscular injection.

Results of the Right Treatment by the Right Route in the Right Dose for the Right Patient

Our sergeant felt enormously better. His hematocrit rose like gangbusters to 52%, and his nervous system signs and symptoms disappeared. His pecker worked just fine, and he no longer felt the nurses, technicians, and dieticians were out to kill him. In fact, the opposite was true. He felt they were saints, and he felt his doctor walked on water. Thus, we have another case of a doctor playing God. When a doctor friend of mine got to heaven, he saw some guy walking around with a stethoscope and asked Saint Peter who that was. "That's God. He likes to play doctor."

Sorry. That was a bad joke.

I was younger then. I felt an intense exhilaration, like a conquering general after a great battle. There have been too many saves and too many patients for me to have the same feelings now. But I still like the idea of curing people and the satisfaction I suspect few people besides physicians ever get. The greatest joy of all is to see someone who had been very sick and considered hopeless walk out of the hospital.

Two years later, our sergeant returned to clinic with the same condition all over again. He had decided he was cured and didn't see any reason to continue the B12 injections every month. He felt fine for over a year despite no injections, so he concluded that he didn't need them. What he didn't know is the liver stores B12 for a time, and then when stored B12 is used up, the pernicious anemia roars back. When the pernicious anemia returned, so did the nervous system signs and symptoms, including the malfunctioning pecker.

Result: Back on the Intramuscular B12—Back to Normal

The sergeant's paranoia proves specific deficiencies can cause signs and symptoms considered characteristic of psychiatric disease. Organic disease can produce signs and symptoms of psychiatric disease. This important point is illustrated by some patient stories to follow, but first a sidebar about nitrous oxide and vitamin B12, since we are on the subject of that important vitamin.

Patients 3, 4, & 5
Dentists Arrive in Clinic

Three dentists arrived in wheelchairs. All had read an article somewhere about the toxic nature of nitrous oxide. All were inhaling nitrous (also known as laughing gas) as a recreation. One of them had his nurse strap it on during lunch so he could operate in the afternoon with a buzz on. The trouble with nitrous oxide is it oxidizes the cobalt at the center of vitamin B12 (remember cobalt is there at the center?) and that makes the B12 ineffective. So, with enough exposure, all inhaling enough nitrous oxide will develop combined systems disease as if they were B12 deficient.

Treatment did improve our dentists, but not that much. Once this kind of nervous system damage occurs over years, it is hard to reverse. The same problem occurs in people with anorexia nervosa after they get nitrous oxide. Their B12 reserves are low because of malnutrition, and therefore the nitrous has a devastating effect. This side effect of nitrous oxide is now generally known, even by surgeons, and the immediate administration of B12 saves the patients from serious disability.

Patients 6 & 7
Priests Who Needed to Remember Something Important

In 1969, I set up a memory clinic at the Neurological Institute. Neurologists knew about the clinic and referred patients with memory problems to me for diagnosis and treatment. Since the clinic was financed by the Gorney-Raisback Fellowship in Human Memory under the auspices of the New York Academy of Medicine, no patients were charged. Consequently, the clinic was very busy. Among the first patients were two priests. They had received what they thought was a rather generous cash donation and decided to celebrate with a bender. Bender is the Irish term for heavy drinking. During the bender, for reasons known only to God, the money apparently disappeared, for when they awoke sober the following morning, the money was missing, and the priests couldn't recall where it went. A detailed search of the Rectory with the help of two housekeepers failed to find the loot. So, the priests were here in clinic hoping for a miracle because the usual dictum at the time was that memories lost under such circumstances are never recovered.

Me: "Fathers, and did you not give the holy water a try or pray to the Virgin Mary for assistance?"

The priests stared at me in stony silence, daggers in their eyes and frowns on their faces.

Me: "Sorry, Fathers, that was just a joke, a stupid joke. Please accept my sincere apology.

"Actually, you're in luck. Chances are you will find out what happened. Human memory is state dependent. What you need to do is get into the brain state you were in during the bender, and the odds are you will recall the events that happened at the time. Context is important and so is mood. My advice is one of you get drunk again with the same whiskey, in the same room in the rectory, at the same time of day, wearing the same clothes. Try to get into the same celebratory mood and mode that you were in when you started the bender. Take in the drinks at the same rate as you did before. Simulate the bender as close as possible. After the playback, report to me what happened."

Result

When priest A was sufficiently drunk, he remembered they decided to hide the money so it could not be stolen. The $5,000 was in the light fixture in the bedroom, a hiding place that may have been suggested by the movie *The Lost Weekend*.

Astronauts train several hundred thousand times here on Earth to do a task they are supposed to do in space. But when they get up there, they often have great difficulty figuring out what to do or even how to start. Only with detailed coaching can they get the job done. When the same astronauts return to Earth, they breeze through the same task. Similarly, if the astronauts learn something in space, they have trouble recalling it when they are back from space, but when reinserted into zero gravity, no problem. Mice and rats who learn a maze under the influence of alcohol, curare, or barbiturate, can't run the maze so well unless their brains are adjusted to the brain state during which learning actually took place. Pianists know full well about state-dependent learning and try to practice under conditions that simulate as closely as possible the playback conditions they will experience in the concert hall.

By the way, dear reader, what is your diagnosis? What caused the loss of memory in these priests? I hope you are still with me, and I pause for reply.

Diagnosis is binge drinking (five or more drinks in a two-hour period) with alcohol-induced blackout. Blackouts are common in heavy drinking and may exist en bloc as it did here with the priests in which they recalled nothing, or there may be partial memories of events that happened. Blackouts are dangerous because people wake up with no memory. Think how disconcerting it is for a woman to awake with a vagina full of goo and not remember how, why, or with whom she had sex. Think how disconcerting it is for a man to wake with his penis covered with fecal material. Ugh! Thus, one of the many side effects of blackouts is sexually transmitted disease. One of the many side effects of binge drinking is also serious injury or even death. The reason binge drinking is defined as five or more drinks in a two-hour period is that during that time the liver is unable to keep up the detox of the alcohol, so blood alcohol levels rise quickly, and brain function is significantly impaired.

Lesson: Binge drinking is bad.

Organic Disease Simulating Mental Illness

Patient Robert
New York State Psychiatric Institute

His first name was Robert, but I find it irritating I can't recall his last name. It wasn't Lenin or Lenski, but it was something like that. Russian sounding. He was an in-patient in the New York Psychiatric Institute because of episodes of extreme impulse control disorder. For no apparent reason, he would clutch his head, complain of severe headache, and then proceed to crash and trash anything and everything in his room. Sometimes during the episodes, he would urinate on the floor, bed, or furniture as he saw fit and wasn't ashamed of this one bit. Sometimes during the episodes, he remained silent, his legs would weaken, and he would descend to the floor, but he would continue moving forward as if he were a Russian dancer, not quite hitting the floor with his bottom and looking like he should be in a movie about drunk Russian men showing off at one of those all-night drinking parties. During one attack, I held his left hand as he descended and walked with him as he continued to move forward like a spider or a crab.

The diagnosis was easy because he had, on examination of the back of the eye with the ophthalmoscope, severe papilledema. Psychiatric disease couldn't produce that finding. The papilledema meant Robert had increased intracranial pressure and had to have an organic cause, not a psychological cause, for his problem.

Diagnosis: Colloid Cyst of the Third Ventricle

The pneumoencephalogram (a terrible, painful test now replaced by CAT scan) showed a colloid cyst of the third ventricle. The cyst was mobile enough to episodically block the aqueduct that drains spinal fluid from the third ventricle. When the aqueduct was blocked, the spinal fluid would build up under pressure, the lateral ventricles of the brain would expand, and the patient's frontal lobes would be adversely affected, and a headache would follow. Cortical spinal fibers from the motor cortex of the brain to the legs travel close by so that when the lateral ventricles dilate enough, the patient's legs would get weak. Consult professor Google if you are interested in knowing more about impulse control syndromes and look up the interesting and famous case of Phineas P. Gage, a sweet nice man who turned into a monster when his left frontal lobe was damaged during a rock blasting accident by an iron rod that passed completely through his skull.

Under the supervision of Lester Mount, the neurosurgical residents removed the cyst, and Robert returned to normal—no more headaches—no more attacks.

Other patients whom I have taken care of who had psychiatric manifestations of neurological disease are too numerous to mention. But one that stands out was a

16-year-old woman who was having mood episodes during which she would suddenly shiver and then cry out, "A big black man is coming up behind me to get me. He's coming. He's coming! He is going to choke me! Help!" The usual mood alteration lasted two minutes and 37 seconds and occurred 16 to 27 times a day.

The electroencephalogram showed seizure discharges in the anterior tip of the right temporal lobe during attacks and some seizure spikes between attacks. The arteriogram and the brain scan showed a tumor there (in the tip of the right temporal lobe). The tumor was easily removed. It was a benign oligodendroglioma. After surgery, the patient had no more episodes.

The facts show nervous system disease can mimic psychiatric disorder. What about vice-versa? Can psychiatric disease mimic neurological disease?

You bet. Consider the illustrations that follow.

Tableau Sixteen:
Psychiatric Conditions Simulating Neurological Conditions

Uncontrolled and Uncontrollable Seizures in a Teenaged Girl

The patient was a 14-year-old girl from Louisiana who had been in and out of hospitals in Louisiana for treatment of grand mal seizures. In fact, she had spent most of the year in three different hospitals. Multiple treatment programs using all of the known antiepileptic drugs of the era had failed to control the attacks. She was referred to me in the hope I could do something. The original idea was I might try to control the seizures with a ketogenic diet. The ketogenic diet, in those days, was used exclusively to control seizures in children who did not respond to other treatments. It is still used in children and is effective. In my era, for unknown reasons, the ketogenic diet was not generally considered a proper treatment for adults with seizures.

Applying the same diet to an adolescent adult seemed reasonable in view of the super-refractory seizures the patient had. Because of the nature of the diet and the possible complications thereof, the patient is best admitted to the hospital during induction of the ketogenic diet.

On neurological examination, the patient was normal, as was every blood test I could think of.

There was something unusual about the records that came from Louisiana: the electroencephalogram was normal while she was not having a seizure, and there was no record of an electroencephalogram during a seizure. About this, I called the referring neurologist, who told me there was no record during an attack because every time they tried to get a recording during an attack the patient's flailing arms pulled off the electrodes.

So, in the electroencephalogram lab, I told the technicians to run in as soon as an attack occurred, and I told them to hold the patient's arms and legs down on the bed so she could not pull off the electrodes. The techs did as they were told.

The EEG during the attack was normal! That meant the attacks were not real. They were feigned. She was pretending to have seizures. But why?

She came to my office. I told her why I knew the seizures were not real, and I told her I knew she had a reason for pretending she had seizures. And I knew it was a very important reason. I told her I would sit there with her until she got up and left or she told me what was bothering her.

135

She was sitting in such a way that my office clock was behind her, and I could see the clock and note the passage of time. And so, we sat there, the two of us looking at each other in silence. One hour and 47 minutes into the mission, she began to cry, and then she told the whole story, showing once again the advantage conferred by low-tech patient-doctor communication.

Her father had been raping her. The way she got out of the nasty situation was to be admitted to a hospital for control of seizures. Rape is a felony, and this rape was all the more egregious because it involved incest. The social worker found out the mother was an accomplice and had full knowledge of what was going on. The mother would leave the house to shop whenever the father wanted to do the nasty. The law comes down hard on this crime. The father went in for eight years, and mom was committed to an asylum in Louisiana. The patient had ambivalent feelings about betraying her father and mother and causing the trouble. The girl also became psychotic and had to be admitted to an asylum. This is not unusual. Often an entire family is crazy, not just one person.

On the other hand, some people are really crazy as the cases that follow indicate.

Tableau Seventeen:

The Truly Psychotic are Different from You and Me

Columbia-Presbyterian Medical Center
Patient with Paranoia

"What brings you to clinic?" I asked, and he said, "The A train."

"Sorry. I meant why did you come to psychiatry clinic?"

"I don't know. The triage nurse downstairs in the emergency room sent me. All I wanted from her was the answer to a simple question. Instead, she sent me up here to psychiatry."

"What's the question?"

"I want to know why people say gas-o-lean instead of gas-o-line."

"Excuse me," says I, "I want to consult one of the doctors in the hall, and I will be right back."

I closed the door and found the attending psychiatrist who was supervising clinic. He was young, just out of residency, and dressed in a black, three-piece suit with a maroon tie.

"There is nothing wrong with my patient. He just had a question. He wanted to know why people say gas-o-lean and not gas-o-line. To me, it sounds like a good question, and I guess it is just social convention."

The psychiatrist stroked his chin, rolled his eyes, then put on a face of deep concern. "Holy cow. He is questioning the whole structure of our language, the social conventions by which we communicate and relate to each other. He must be schizophrenic. I better go in there and handle him with you. Probably he is paranoid as hell. I'll bring out the paranoia with a few questions. Why did he come to clinic?"

"The triage nurse sent him. But when I first asked him what brought him to clinic, he said the A train."

"The A train! Sweet Jesus! Concrete thinking! You can't get any more concrete than that. He must be schizophrenic."

Me: "Mr. X, this is Doctor Y, who is helping me in clinic. Doctor Y would like to ask you some questions."

Psychiatrist: "Did anything unusual happen today?"

Patient: "Yes. This morning there was a thermonuclear attack on the Bronx. The Russians destroyed the Bronx, and all the people except me were killed. I alone have survived."

Psychiatrist: "Anything else?"

Patient: "Some people moved my Volkswagen to the other side of the street and reversed the direction, so it is facing the wrong way. How they lifted it, I don't know. There must have been several guys because it's pretty heavy."

Psychiatrist: "Why would they move your car?"

Patient: "People are after me."

Psychiatrist: "People are after you?"

Patient: "I don't know why. But they are."

Out in the hall again, the psychiatrist said, "Notice the paranoia. Schizophrenics are people who are trying to make up for a weak ego by pretending in their own minds they are very special. Notice he is so special he alone survived a thermonuclear attack on the Bronx. People are after him because he is special, a VIP of sorts. By the way, some paranoids are justified by their ideas. So always check for the reality. In this case, we would have heard the boom if the Russians attacked. And the radio would have told us about the attack. So, we are sure this man is under the delusion the Russians attacked the Bronx when we know they didn't. The Russians may attack tomorrow, but for sure they did not attack the Bronx today. That is just a crazy delusion.

"But keep in mind sometimes, what sounds paranoid is real. Hemingway got three years of psychotherapy because he felt the C.I.A. was following him. Hemingway couldn't shake the idea, and the psychotherapy didn't help. But it turns out the C.I.A was following him. During that time, they thought he was a commie, and they wanted to keep their eye on him. We know this is true from the freedom of information act.

"Start your patient on Thorazine, 50 mg once a day. Next week, check him in clinic. This will be a good patient for you to learn from. My prediction is next week he will be normal. That is the benefit of treating schizophrenia early. That will prove that psychiatrists do good and can do good."

Sure enough, next week came, and the patient was normal. He told me he must have been crazy to think that the Russians attacked, and he was crazy to think people moved his car. They did not. "Many thanks, Doc. I feel enormously better. The reason people say gas-o-lean is everyone says it that way, and the way you get to be understood is by following the crowd."

Thinking about paranoia reminds me of two other patients similarly afflicted: Joyce and Joe Lee. Basically, there are two types of lunatics: the harmless lunatic and the dangerous lunatic. Joyce and Joe Lee were the dangerous type.

Baylor College of Medicine
Joyce

In clinic one Thursday afternoon, I looked out from the examining room and thought I saw a familiar face among the 50 or so people waiting. I couldn't place the face until Luisa, the nurse, put the woman in an exam room. The patient was Joyce, the woman who cuts my hair at a salon called Gentlemen's Choice, NASA Road One and El Camino Real in Clear Lake City.

"Joyce, what are you doing here?"

"I had to see someone about the voice of God. You are the only doctor I trust."

"Voice of God?"

"When I cut hair, I hear the voice of God telling me to stab the scissors into the customer's neck."

"Joyce, did you ever hear the voice tell you to stab me?"

"Last time it was very loud and commanded me to stab you. Why would God tell me to do that?"

"Did the voice ever tell you to stab my son, Craig?"

"Him too. I know it's wrong to stab someone. But if God commands it, wouldn't it be OK?"

"Joyce, that is not the voice of God. And it is not OK to stab someone. That voice means you are insane, but part of you is sane. That's why you came for help. Part of you knows it is wrong. The sane part of you is reaching out asking for help."

Joyce glowered at me. "I'm insane because I hear the voice of God? Lots of saints have heard the voice of God. Why would that make me insane and them sane?"

Joyce had a point here, but the Diagnostic and Statistical Manual of Psychiatric conditions does make an exception for religion. In fact, part of the definition of a delusion is: a false belief not amenable to logical persuasion and not part of a religious system.

"God wouldn't tell you to do an evil thing. The voice is not the voice of God. Hearing the voice and thinking it is really from God, means there is a defect in your ability to tell the real from the fake. Because the voice is telling you to hurt someone, we have to protect the public from you. And we have to protect you from doing a criminal act. We have to lock you up until you get over this illness. You need a rest."

"You think I'm crazy!"

"Nope! Joyce, I don't think you're crazy. I know you're crazy. Because you're crazy, we need to put you in a safe place so you can't hurt people. This is required by the law. The nurses will get things ready for you to go to Rusk State Hospital. The doctors there will help you. I hope after a long rest and good treatment you will recover."

Notice how Joyce confirms the theories about the two interpreters of the state of mind. Interpreter one, in her case, makes her hear the voice of God telling her to harm the client. Interpreter two tells her that is not right, and she should talk to Doctor Patten about this. Doubting the craziness is considered a good sign. Enough doubt is in there to give reality a toehold. Hence, Joyce's prognosis is better than the prognosis for most paranoid schizophrenics.

Joyce spent four years in the loony bin and returned after her recovery to ask to have her license to cut hair restored. What do you think, dear reader? Should she get her license back or not?

I pause for reply.

Answer: of course not! Are you crazy? And you can bet when I go for a haircut these days, I keep the haircutter under close observation.

Lesson: Mental illness is real and has to be dealt with realistically. If they look like they might hurt themselves or others, they have to be stopped. It is an important duty of physicians to put the dangerous mental patients in an asylum.

The Truly Psychotic are Different from You and Me

The next patient, Joe Lee, was even sicker than Joyce.

Baylor College of Medicine
Joe Lee

Joe had a routine case of peripheral neuropathy with weakness of arms and legs and sensory loss in a glove-and-stocking distribution. Most neurologists would not approve of how I handle patients like this, but what I did was prescribe every vitamin known to affect nerve function. That is my vitamin cocktail. Joe responded, and the neuropathy disappeared. No tests. No biopsies. No hospitalization. Just vitamins. There is a population in Texas malnourished and vitamin deficient. They will recover from their nerve disease with tincture of time and vitamins.

There was another thing on physical exam that I forgot to mention. It might have been an indication of the trouble to come, or it might have just been a tattoo. Joe had on the surface skin over his right deltoid muscle a tattoo that read: "Fock it All." The tattoo may have been meant to display some other four-letter word which the tattoo artist did not know how to spell. Anyway— "Fock it all" is what the tattoo read.

Four months after his complete recovery from his neuropathy at 4:12 p.m. Thursday afternoon, Joe called. "Doctor Patten, I saw you and nurse Luisa kill that old woman in that shed in northern Harris County. So, I went to the DA to tell them, and they threw me out. So, I went to the FBI to tell them about the murder, and they threw me out. So now I have to take justice into my own hands and come and kill you and Luisa. I am calling to tell you this, so you know why I have to kill you."

Before I could say anything, Joe hung up.

We took Polaroid pictures of every patient who came to clinic. Nurse Luisa fished Joe's picture out of the file, made copies, and distributed them to everyone she could think of including Methodist security and the Houston Police. The police said that I should carry a gun, even though it was illegal at the time. They thought I had a good reason, and if something happened and I had to shoot Joe, there wouldn't be much trouble for me as it would have been justified self-defense. They also said it is a crime to threaten to kill someone, and Joe would be arrested when found.

I decided not to carry a gun because Jesus said, "He who lives by the sword dies by the sword." By this reasoning, if I didn't carry a gun, I wouldn't get shot. Pop, my father and at one time the District Attorney of Queens, had a license to carry but didn't for the same reason. It worked for him. He died at the breakfast table just after giving his usual speech: "Another day and another step closer to the grave."

The Police Stop Joe

That afternoon, the Houston police arrested Joe in front of the Methodist Hospital on the east side of Main Street. Joe was carrying a shotgun, which the police took away. They brought him to the emergency room, where he stayed with a police guard. Joe mentioned the delusion he had seen Luisa and me kill a woman. So, psychiatry consultation was requested. While waiting for the psychiatrist, the cop left Joe for a few minutes to go to the loading dock to smoke a cigarette. When he returned, Joe was gone.

That night, Joe's father called. "Doctor Patten, I have bad news. Joe broke into our home and took my automatic rifle. He said he was headed your way to kill you."

The next call was from Joe himself. "Just calling to let you know I'm coming to get you. You gave me the slip last time, but you won't escape again."

The Houston police again arrested Joe in front of the Methodist Hospital. They took away his father's rifle and made sure Joe got to see the psychiatrist. A psychotic who is a danger to himself or others had to be committed. Joe spent the next four years in Rusk State hospital.

Lesson: That was the old days when it was easy to get these dangerous nut cases off the street and into the hospital. Now I am informed there is a four-month waiting list to get into Rusk. If we don't get the dangerous lunatics off the streets and into the nut hut, they will cause trouble, lots of trouble.

When Joe got out, he called and apologized for his behavior. "Jesus, I must have been some sick cookie. I am so sorry. I know you and Luisa wouldn't kill anyone. Please take me back as your patient."

"Joe, if I ever see you again, I'll call the cops."

Joyce and Joe were psychotic and dangerous. They are interesting, but the neurotics are more interesting. Some types of neurotic disease simulate neurologic conditions.

Neurosis Simulating Neurological Disease

Baylor College of Medicine
Before We Get to the Next Patient, a Primer on Psychoanalysis

Two great systems of ideas help us understand human nature: literature and psychoanalysis. Psychoanalysis makes two claims: it is a science, and it is a method. As a theory of mental life, it is especially useful to cure neurosis as will be demonstrated in the case studies that follow. Both the science and the method base themselves on a few fundamental discoveries, which seem trite to us now, but were not trivial or trite 80 years ago. Among them are: the unconscious, the mechanisms of repression, the formative power of early experiences in life, dreams as an expression of fears and desires, and, more generally, the frightening power of emotions and the irrational in determining human behavior for good or for evil.

Nurse Z

A nurse came to the emergency room assisted by her neighbor. The nurse had suddenly gone blind and asked the neighbor to take her to the ER. There, she asked for me to take care of her. The examination showed she had a normal nervous system, including pupillary reactions to light. When I faced her to the wall and asked her to keep walking, she stopped just as her nose touched the wall and went no further. Obviously, she didn't want to hurt her nose. This was good evidence she could see, but for some important psychological reason she did not want to think or admit to her conscious mind she could see. This serious state was known in the old days as hysterical blindness or conversion hysteria. The idea was the patient needed to convert an unwanted idea into a physical symptom. The unwanted material had to be hidden from consciousness because facing it would produce too much anxiety. Thus, the neuroses were mental tricks (called mental mechanisms) to reduce anxiety. Usually, the physical symptom has symbolic significance. A neurosis is, therefore, another way to cope with the troubles of a difficult situation in a troubled world. The problem is the neurosis often wastes time and energy, and it almost never solves the underlying psychological problem. Hence, the need to face the facts and get the buried (now unconscious) material out in the open where it can be managed better.

Patients with conversions are not concerned about their plight. If you or I had suddenly gone blind, we would be very upset. People with psychological blindness seem pretty much indifferent to the blindness as was this nurse. The lack of concern is known in psychiatric circles as "La belle indifference." My theory is they are not concerned because at some level they know they are not really blind.

Handling patients with neuroses is like working through a detective novel. There were three clues as to the cause of the nurse's problem: 1. She is not blind for a

147

physical reason. 2. She is blind for a psychological reason. 3. She saw something she didn't want to see. How can a blind nurse see what she saw? In other words, the blindness is the reason she is using to tell herself she didn't see what she saw. Get it? If not, read on.

The key to understanding her case was to take her back to the exact time and place of the blindness. In this setting, place memory is much more important than time memory. In humans, place memory is much more solid than time memory. So, when you can't recall something, think of where not when.

"Where were you and what were you doing and why were you doing it when you went blind?"

The nurse and I had a talk session every day for two weeks. Suddenly, she screamed and beat the chair with her fists. She was no longer blind! She saw clearly. A miracle? Nope. She remembered she was looking for a paperclip and opened the middle draw of her husband's desk in his study. There she saw pictures of her best girlfriend in many sexual positions with her (the nurse's) husband. This was the stuff she didn't want to see, the stuff she repressed into the unconscious.

Abreaction, the necessary devastating correction, followed.

Abreaction is a psychoanalytical term for reliving an experience in order to purge it of its emotional significance and excesses. This type of hypercathected catharsis often involves becoming conscious of repressed emotionally traumatic events.

In 1893, Sigmund Freud came up with the idea that pent-up emotions could be discharged by talking about them. Our nurse did more than talk to discharge her pent-up emotions. She divorced her husband.

Two years later, they remarried, and two years after that, they divorced again.

It was puzzling why the nurse's husband, a physician, would leave incriminating pictures in his unlocked desk drawer and more puzzling that a wife would rummage through that draw looking for a paperclip. There is more to this story than meets the eye, much more. There usually is. This case, Freud would have had a field day. Human beings—trés compliqué.

Patients like this nurse with functional neurological symptoms are a challenge for neurologists. Among neurologists in the United Kingdom, such patients are considered "among the most difficult to help." Among U.S. neurologists, functional neurological conditions are the least liked. I don't know why. Most of them should be amenable to treatment if treated before the functional disability becomes an ingrained habit of the brain. Diagnostic and Statistical Manual (DSM) V changes DMS IV criteria for functional illness by eliminating criterion B (the positive identification of a psychological disorder) and criterion C (the condition should not be deliberately feigned). Thus, the diagnosis is easier to justify.

Most studies report lack of recovery in one-half to two-thirds of patients. That is bad. Factors contributing to the failure to improve include negative expectations, denial of psychological factors, and receipt of health-related financial benefits. My own take is most current neurologists don't have the interest, time, or skill to cure such patients, and that's too bad because most of these patients might be curable either by short-term psychotherapy, behavior deconditioning, or strong suggestion; one, two, three of those treatments or any combination thereof. As an "old school neurologist," I liked taking care of these patients. Nowadays, I think, this group of patients is underserved. We old school neurologists, in order to get board certified, had to pass written, oral, and practical examinations in both neurology and psychiatry. Somewhere along the line, I think the rules changed, and neurologists are not examined in psychiatry and psychiatrists are not examined in neurology. That's a shame. A good neurologist should know psychiatry and vice-versa. Sigmund Freud was both a neurologist and a psychiatrist. He was trained in neurology by Charcot, one of the most famous neurologists of all time. And Charcot was keen on treating not only patients with organic diseases of the nervous system but patients with neuroses as well. After headache, functional neurological disorders (conversions reactions, dissociative nonepileptic seizures, functional movement disorders) are the most common reason for outpatient neurological consultation (reference: Neurology 2014;83:2299-2301).

Notice how analysis of the nurse-patient resulted in the blindness going away. Freud said psychotics were unanalyzable because they couldn't distinguish between fantasy and reality, and analysis works precisely on that distinction. That's why the psychotics get the drugs or the nut hut (insane asylum), and the neurotics get the talk treatment. Freud also said the Irish were unanalyzable. He didn't explain why. As an Irishman, I can affirm we Irish think we are unanalyzable. We Irish are all sane and, therefore, don't need and won't cooperate with analysis. And that reminds me of my Irish aunt and her problem.

My Aunt Joan Patten

Aunt Joan was the youngest of the aunts on my father's side. Sunday nights would often find her driving me back to Columbia College. Along the way, we talked and became good friends and confidants. Most of us called Aunt Joan "Joan" because she was young like us, her nephews. Joan was the aunt who supplied the Parliament cigarettes for us kids to smoke in the basement. In many ways she was a kid, only a little older than we were.

One Sunday, Joan said she was having a gigantic problem getting into elevators and riding the subway. Every time she tried to get into the elevator or a subway car, she would start to tremble, get short of breath, break out into a sweat, and sometimes collapse. Joan now had to drive herself into Manhattan, pay an outrageous price to park, and climb 57 flights of stairs to get to her job as a secretary.

Analysis: Joan has an intrapsychic conflict. She is managing the conflict by projecting the conflict to the outside world. In this case: elevators and subway trains, which she can manage by avoiding elevators and subways. Joan is paying a price for this kind of neurotic adaptation and is not happy about the situation. So, the real deal is to find the source of the conflict and resolve it. Resolving the conflict will make the neurosis unnecessary, and it will therefore disappear. Usually, the conflict is about sex.

The Conflict

Joan was a good Catholic. She had a nice boyfriend who wanted to have sex but who didn't want to get married. Joan loved this guy but didn't want to have sex with him unless they were married, as unmarried sex would be a mortal sin. As her nephew, I didn't feel it was my place to advise her about how to resolve the conflict, so I referred her to Doctor Ryan, a friend of mine at the New York Psychiatric Institute.

Joan called to tell me what happened. "Ryan listened to my story for 10 minutes. Then he stood up and pointed his finger at me and said: "Joan, screw him or leave him."

"Are you going to follow Ryan's advice?"

"Of course. Do you think I'm crazy? He charged me $125. I am going to do what he said. In fact, I have already done it. Today, I told Robert he either marries me or leaves. He left. Good riddance."

"And?"

"No more trouble with subways or elevators. It's a miracle. Made a believer of me. Ryan saved me lots of parking money and lots of time. His fee was well worth it."

Joan's experience also made a believer of me. Although her story may seem to be simplistic and unconvincing, that's the way it happened.

> **Lesson:** Sometimes, people have simple problems simply solved.

When I told Joan's story to Robert Williams, the chief of psychiatry at Baylor College of Medicine, he nodded and said, "cases like hers made a believer of me."

Baylor College of Medicine
Mrs. ABC

This 45-year-old woman was sent from a small hick town in north Texas for evaluation and treatment of paralysis of both legs. The paralysis had come on one night as she was returning from choir practice. She had been in a wheelchair for the last four years. On examination, her nervous system was normal. She did not seem particularly concerned about the paralysis and said she had made an adjustment to being a cripple. "But if you, Doctor Patten, can make me whole again, please do."

Analysis: conversion reaction involving paralysis of both legs. Situation caused by some kind of intrapsychic conflict, which might come out with talk treatment. No luck on the talking, so I hypnotized her. (There was a course at Columbia's Medical School that I took. I held a certificate in clinical hypnosis and my hospital privileges at Methodist Hospital included hypnosis.)

She went into a nice trance with a simple Braid induction. Taking her back to the day and the place that the paralysis started revealed she had been running home. Along the way, in the dark, she fell over a toy wagon left on the sidewalk. Both knees were abraded with the fall and then and there she was unable to move her legs.

"Why were you running?"

Abreaction. A big one.

She was running back home from church. That night, her minister asked her to stay after choir practice, and one thing led to another, and he raped her. Whether he raped her or not is debatable. It may have been a mutual consent or part rape and part consent. Who knows? She liked thinking it was a rape because that put the blame on the minister and not on her. So what! If that belief made her more comfortable and didn't hurt the minister, so what! The key point was the emotional event was now out in open consciousness, and after a while, it was reasonable and expected and probable she would walk again.

The next day, she got out of the wheelchair and walked! The nurses and the medical students thought a miracle had happened. Indeed, it did look like a miracle.

She left the hospital recovered. Needless to say, many patients from that little hick town in North Texas came to consult me about their illnesses. I wish I could have been as effective with them as I had been with her.

I couldn't think of anything to do about the minister. He might be a danger to other women. Who knows? Not knowing what to do about him, I did nothing. Sorry.

Speak memory. Just thinking of the emergency room and the blind nurse reminds me of two other patients that I met in the emergency room.

The Young Man Who Arrived in the ER in Coma and the Electrical Engineer Who Couldn't Remember He Ate Dinner

Columbia-Presbyterian Medical Center
Young Man from the Car Crash

This 23-year-old man was carried in by the police who had extracted him from a crashed car. The car had been headed north on the West Side Highway when it veered off course and crashed into a tree.

On examination, the patient was in coma and had no responses to external stimuli, including pinprick and strong pinches. His pupils were very small, pinpoint, and that made it difficult to see into the back of the eye with the ophthalmoscope. Because of the difficulty seeing the fundus (the back of the eye), the medical resident called for a neurological consult—namely me. The condition of the back of the eye is important in the intelligent appraisal of any person in coma because any kind of increase in pressure on the brain could show up as a swelling of the optic nerve that can be seen with the ophthalmoscope.

"No sign of intracranial pressure, but the pupils are so small I can't tell if they react to light," I told the medical resident. Then I noticed a vein in the left antecubital fossa (elbow region) was bleeding. "Did anyone draw blood?"

No one remembered drawing blood. The other thing was respirations were only three breaths a minute, a value below normal. Normal breathing should be about 12, sometimes as much as 16 times a minute.

Thus, putting the clues together: slow breathing, pinpoint pupils (very small pupils are characteristic of morphine-like drugs including heroin), vein bleeding from the left arm (the favorite spot for drug addicts to use), and coma. I concluded this was a drug overdose, probably due to New York City's favorite drug at the time—heroin. Is it still the favorite?

"Hey, let's give some Naline to wake him up."

Naline is the antidote for opiate poisoning. It is effective and works right away. The drawback is that if the coma is due to some other cause, the Naline might make the coma worse. The other name for Naline is nalorphine or chemically N-allyl-nor-morphine. It is a mixed opioid agonist-antagonist that acts on two receptors in the brain. It is antagonistic to the mu receptor and stimulates the kappa. If this man's coma is due to heroin stimulation of the mu receptor, then the Naline would reverse the coma, and the patient would wake up to tell us what was what.

The medical resident was underwhelmed. He was one of those bread and butter doctors who were fine for the easy cases but had trouble handling the hard cases, the cases you never read about in a medical textbook, the cases like the one we were dealing with right then, the cases that required creative thinking.

Medical Resident: "No way. Are you out of your mind? The cops just brought him in from a crash. His car was totaled. The coma is due to trauma, and Naline will make it worse, possibly bump him off. Sometimes you neurologists can't see the obvious."

"How about a trial of a small dose of Naline? If the coma gets worse, we will know something. If it gets better, we will know something."

The medical resident injected a small dose of Naline, five milligrams.

We waited.

Two minutes later, nothing had changed except respirations were now six per minute and not three. To me, this was evidence of response to the Naline. To the medical resident, it was of no significance whatsoever.

"The way we know something for sure is by measurement. "Measurement began our might," said the Irish poet Yeats. The way to know something for sure is to measure it. In this case, the respirations went up from three to six. That is a 100% improvement, strong evidence, in my view, this is coma due to overdose. "So, let's give the right dose of Naline and wake him up."

"No way! The Naline test was negative," said the medical resident shaking his head in the nugatory mode.

"Be reasonable. We have five clues this is an overdose: slow breathing, faster breathing after Naline, pinpoint pupils, vein bleed, and coma. The only thing that doesn't make sense, that doesn't add up is the car crash. How that fits in, I don't know. But there is no external evidence of trauma except this bleeding vein, which looks like it was punctured with a needle."

The medical resident didn't agree and remained intransigent about more Naline, so I accepted the patient as my patient and agreed to admit him to my neurology ward service and take care of him there. Once the patient was transferred to me, the medical resident had nothing more to say, for now, I was in charge of the case, and now I had the say-so about what to do."

The Young Man Who Arrived in the ER in Coma and the Electrical Engineer

So, I said to the nurse, "More Naline. 15 milligrams this time."

The patient got the next dose of Naline. Two minutes later, he sat up, looked around, and asked, "What the hell? Where am I?"

Ah! Naline. I love it. Now they are giving it away so addicts can themselves reverse an overdose and save the health care system time, energy, and money. It should also be available as an over-the-counter agent so anyone can buy it and keep it around in case of need.

His Story

He was tired of being a drug addict and decided to end it all by injecting a massive dose of heroin while driving at full speed. That was very inconsiderate of him, wouldn't you say, and indicated he was a danger both to himself and others and needed admission to the New York State Psychiatric Institute, where he would spend the next few months awaiting trial for his crimes, and where the shrinks would detox him and make an attempt at rehab.

News: the police found a note on the front seat of the wrecked car. It read: "I am sick of the drug sceen (sic) and I will end (it) by killing myself."

The police said, "This guy is a bad hombre. A God-damn-fuck-up-son-of-a-bitch-bastard. He will get lots of time to think things over. The car was hot."

New York's finest don't like jerks who crash their cars on purpose endangering themselves and the public. I agreed with them. This patient was a disgusting nothing and should be put away for quite a while. No, change that. That was unkind. If we knew enough about this young man and his situation, we might be more understanding and forgiving. He is a human just like us and needs help. No question he needs jail time. But perhaps he can be rehabilitated. Comprendre tout, c'est tout pardonner. That's French: to understand everything, is to forgive everything. Judge not that you be not judged.

Later, the patient's story changed. The drugs were part of the scene, but the main problem was: "My gal done left me and ain't come back."

Even as I write this, many men for lack of love alone are making friends with death just as this guy did.

Almost always, the problem is something deeper than just drugs. Benn Crader, the scientist in Saul Bellow's 1987 novel, *More Die of Heartbreak*, states what we know from science about the troubles modernity has brought to the world must be taken seriously, "But," Crader says, "I think more die of heartbreak."

Pain, discomfort, or just plain yearning make people reach for drugs. The deep question is whether we can look at our drug users and abusers with compassion and infuse its management with mercy.

The Electrical Technician

Two weeks later, there was another consult in the same room as the suicidal drug addict. This patient was more interesting. The consultation request was to rule out nervous system disease for clearance to admit to psychiatry.

Ruling out nervous system disease is, of course, not possible, as most people have something wrong with their nervous system. Those who think they don't have something wrong with their nervous system just have not been examined enough. Psychiatric patients troubled me because every one of them always had, on close examination, definite evidence for brain disease. In fact, my bet is sometime in the distant future, all psychiatric disease will be known to have a physical basis in the malfunction of the nervous system. The cause will be in the nervous system, or it will be an effect originating outside the nervous system, which caused the nervous system to go haywire.

The patient was a 54-year-old man, an electrical technician, who was free of neurological problems according to himself and his wife until that day. At 5 p.m. he returned from work to his apartment. Soon thereafter he poured his usual glass of bourbon whiskey. After he drank the first, he poured another. His wife, seeing the second glass, and knowing he never ever drank more than one bourbon, asked why he was drinking two. Had he had a very difficult day?

The patient looked puzzled and said this was the only drink he poured that day. The telephone rang, and he spoke to his brother about a relative who had died the year before as if that person were still alive. He asked how the deceased was feeling and asked if she had a nice vacation. At that point, the wife, thinking her husband had gone crazy, grabbed the telephone and hung it up in an effort to conceal the insanity from the rest of the world.

Dinner was served, and, reportedly, the patient was very conversational at the table, asking what his son had done in school and what the son did after school. When the meal was finished, the patient retired to the living room and started to read the evening paper. About five minutes after the table had been cleared, he turned down the paper and inquired what was for dinner. When his wife told him that he had already eaten, the patient became angry because he thought his wife was playing a trick on him. "Where's my dinner?" he screamed at her.

Unable to control the situation, the wife called the physician who lived next door. The physician examined the patient briefly and advised that the patient be taken to the emergency room to see a psychiatrist.

At 11 p.m., he was examined by me for the purpose of giving neurological clearance for admission to the Psychiatry Service.

General physical examination was normal, except for bilateral arcus senilis, a white circle around the iris that sometimes indicates a predisposition to cardiovascular disease.

Neurological exam showed a droop of the lower half of the right side of the face, which was subsequently shown to be present on old photographs of the patient. Cranial nerves were normal. He had a normal gait and station. He walked well on toes and heels. He hopped on either foot without difficulty. Arm swing and tandem walking were normal. He stood still in the middle of the room with his eyes closed and did not sway or lose his balance. Results of sensory examination were normal and included light touch, pain, vibration, position sense, two-point discrimination, number writing, cortical localization test, and double simultaneous stimulation. Testing showed excellent fine motor control without even a hint of tremor. Deep tendon reflexes were all normal, and equal bilaterally, and there were no pathological reflexes.

Whew! That was a lot of testing. But remember, this is from a bygone era when physicians actually had the time and energy to do that kind of examination. Indeed, the only abnormalities were on mental status examination.

The patient was awake, alert, and cooperative. He carried on a well-ordered, logical conversation, following his own thoughts and those of others. If distracted, however, he lost the trend of his thought and would often repeat several times whole paragraphs of what he had just spoken about five minutes before. For instance, he knew something was wrong with his memory and wanted to be admitted to the private service under a private doctor, not me, a resident. He, therefore, asked if private beds were available and told me how much he would appreciate having a private doctor. It was explained to him there were no private beds available, and he would have to be admitted to the ward service. He smiled and said, "OK, if you will be my doctor."

A few minutes later, after I left the room and returned, the whole scenario could be reproduced by asking him if he wanted to be admitted as a private patient. The patient would then ask the same questions about the private service and about having a private doctor, with the same intonation and facial gestures as before, as if he had never done these things in his life. From this, it was clear that he did not recall or recognize what had transpired only minutes previously.

At one point, I left the room for five minutes. When I returned, the patient behaved as if he had never seen me before. Formal memory testing showed he was unable to recall verbal or visual material five minutes after distraction. Clues and cues did not help his recall, nor could he identify the correct items from a list. No confabulation occurred. In fact, the patient couldn't recall ever being asked to remember anything.

He was amnesic for the events that happened since the first drink of bourbon. That is, he did not recall pouring the second drink, the call from the relative, eating dinner, or for that matter, coming to the hospital. He did have some kind of vague memory of some tall man looming over him and yelling at him in his apartment. This may have been the physician who was called since that physician is 6 feet 5 inches tall and talks in a loud, rough voice.

The patient knew world events up to about four years ago. And although he gave the present year correctly, he said he was 50 years old when, as mentioned, he was 54. He also thought the dead relative he had asked about on the telephone was still alive and wondered why people got so concerned when he said this. Therefore, he had a retrograde amnesia of at least one year (the year of the relative's death) or even four years since he thought he was 50 and couldn't recall any world event or personal event that happened within the last four years.

The patient knew all the details of his own biography, including his name, address, and telephone number. He wrote the correct formulas for impedance, current, and was able to draw simple electrical diagrams for radios and pentodes. He easily repeated seven digits forward if not distracted. If distracted, he could recall none. On many occasions, he could not repeat any digits backward, even when not distracted. In other words, I would say, "Repeat these numbers forward: 3091," and he did it. "Now say them backward." He couldn't. He was unable to reverse letter sequences as well. Other mental processes that required reorganization also were not possible for him to do. He was not able to do the simplest subtractions like 9 – 3, 3 – 1, 6 – 4, and so forth. He was easily able to spell words forward, but, for the life of him, he could not spell words backward. Example:

The Young Man Who Arrived in the ER in Coma and the Electrical Engineer

Me: "Spell cat."

He: "C-A-T."

Me: "Now spell cat backward."

He: with a puzzled look on his face and shaking his head, he said, "C-A-T is the best I can do."

Me: "That is cat forward. Now do it backward. Start with the last letter and proceed to the beginning of the word."

He: with much mental anguish. "I don't understand what you want."

Me: "Spell the word world."

He: "W-O-R-L-D."

Me: "Correct. Now start with the last letter and work toward the front of the word. So, you will have spelled the word world backward by starting at the last letter and working forward letter by letter to the beginning."

He: after multiple tries, nothing even close.

Despite the disability of spelling backward or subtracting numbers, his use of language was normal. He could write, read, name, repeat, sing in tune, and obey commands like touch your nose, blink your eyes, smile, walk around the room on your toes, and so forth.

OK, dear reader, what should be done? Would you clear him for admission to psychiatry? Would you admit him to neurology? What do you think is happening? Is he sane or crazy?

I pause for reply.

Action

He was admitted to neurology under my care. The attack stopped at 2 a.m. when he began to remember events as they happened and became able to spell forward and backward and do subtractions without difficulty. His mental examination was entirely normal. He was able to remember words, pictures, smells, tastes, touches, and so forth. He could encode memories in any modality without difficulty. This was an amazing recovery without any treatment!

There was no retrograde amnesia. He knew he was 54, he had a fair knowledge of world events that happened during the last four years (as much as the average New Yorker), and he knew his relative had died last year. But he was amnesic for all events that happened during the acute phase of the attack. That is, he recalled nothing from 5 p.m. to 2 a.m., except for the previously mentioned man (probably the doctor next door) standing over him yelling at him.

The blood tests were normal, as were the brain scan and the electroencephalogram. I did a spinal tap and got clear fluid under normal pressure. The laboratory reported normal results on the examination of the fluid.

Under my supervision, the patient drank a half bottle of the same bourbon he had taken two glasses of just prior to his attack. He got drunk, but blood tests every half hour for four hours showed no change in blood sugar, ruling out an alcohol-induced low blood sugar as the cause of his attack. While he was very drunk, he was able to do all of the memory tests, subtractions, word backward, and so forth without difficulty. While drunk, his recent memory was quite good for all modalities. This ruled out alcohol as a cause of the attack.

The patient was followed in clinic. He continued to drink one glass of bourbon daily. He has had no further attacks, nor have there been any signs or symptoms of nervous system or psychiatric disease. He regards the episode as an event isolated from the mainstream of his life; its cause is mysterious to him, as it is to his physicians.

Reader, your diagnosis?

Transient Global Amnesia

The cause of transient global amnesia is not known. Most cases involve a single attack out of the blue with complete recovery, except for amnesia for the events during the attack. The current theory that this is some kind of vascular event involving the sections of the brain concerned with encoding recent memory (CA1 neurons in the hypocamphal part of the temporal lobe of the brain) is unproven. Psychological amnesias are quite different. Psychological amnesias occur after an emotional event, such as the death of a loved one. Patients with psychological amnesias are not concerned about the memory loss. This is the "La Belle Indifference" we talked about in the patients who had conversion reactions. Also, in the psychological amnesias, the patient is often amnesic for their own name, telephone number, and address. The psychological amnesia involves so-called memory loss for distant events of a personal nature. That kind of memory loss is rare in organic diseases of the brain and does not occur in transient global amnesia. Lastly, patients with psychological amnesias never show loss of encoding of recent memories. Patients with psychological amnesias are taciturn and reticent to answer questions because they do not know what an amnesic patient is supposed to say, but if they do cooperate, they will demonstrate a normal memory for recent events. The hallmark feature of transient global amnesia is the inability to do subtractions or to spell backward or do a backward digit span, and those features distinguish the patient with true transient global amnesia from the patient who is psychologically ill. Why patients with global amnesia cannot do these things is not known.

Comment: this is just one of several patients I have seen with this condition. My friend and fellow physician, Pete, called me to ask if I would have lunch with him. The problem was he and I had just had lunch together. "Pete, stay in your lab. I will be right there." Sure enough, Pete was having an attack that lasted eight hours. He recovered completely and has not had another attack in over 20 years. Frances, my tap dance teacher, had an attack during chemotherapy for ovarian cancer. She did not have another attack, despite additional chemo. She recovered just as the others did. We may not know what causes this condition, but we know how to diagnose it, and we know that it will go away without treatment. Recent cases will, no doubt, not be admitted to the hospital or undergo extensive tests.

Reference: Fisher CM Adams RD: *Transient global amnesia.* Acta Neuro Scand 40 (suppl 9):7-83, 1964.

All patients so far, in some manner, presented for medical care. There was one patient I deliberately tried to find, so I could do an experiment. His name was Peter Callas, and his story and the result of the experiment follow.

Tableau Twenty:

The Man Who Pissed in His Pants and Didn't Care

Neurological Institute of New York
Peter Callas

In 1965, a paper appeared in The New England Journal of Medicine describing a new neurological syndrome called normal pressure hydrocephalus. The paper was written by Ray Adams and others. Ray Adams was the professor and chairman of the Department of Neurology at Harvard. You can tell a Harvard man, but you can't tell him much. Thus, a paper coming out of Harvard carried great weight and authority.

A syndrome is a running together of signs or symptoms or both. The pattern of abnormalities can tip off the alert physician about what is causing the patient's difficulties and what to do about them. My genetics professor at Columbia, Theodosius Dobzhansky, used to define a syndrome as "a whore house at the airport" and then laugh his head off at his outstandingly funny side-splitting joke. Theodosius Dobzhansky was even more famous for his quote: "Nothing in biology makes sense except in the light of evolution." That statement is, of course, true. He received the Medal of Science at the White House for his work on human evolution.

But I am getting off the point. Back to the subject: the syndrome of normal pressure hydrocephalus as described by Doctor Adams, like ancient Gaul, consisted of three parts:

- Incontinence of urine.

- A magnetic gait in which the feet appear to be magnetized to the ground. This is just a marked reduction in step height.

- Dementia.

The mnemonic for the syndrome was "wet, wobbly, and wacky."

Because the patients had dementia, they were often misdiagnosed as having Alzheimer's disease (old timer's disease as my Irish aunts used to call it). Because the patients had a gait abnormality, they were often diagnosed as having Parkinson's disease, but unlike the Parks, they had no tremor or rigidity.

Let's go hunting for a patient with this new syndrome. Let's scout out the clinics for someone demented, who doesn't lift his feet, and who pees in his pants. Where should we look? Parkinson's Disease clinic, of course.

In those days, I was gung-ho. So, with the intention of finding the first patient in the City of New York with normal pressure hydrocephalus, I hung out in the Parkinson clinic. The very first day, I found him. I found my man. His name was Peter Callas. He had been demented for four years. He walked as if his feet were glued to the floor, and, according to his wife, he wet his pants several times a day.

There were many details in the transient global amnesia story. Did you get bored? I just wanted to show you how patients were examined in the old days before the scanners took over the universe. In the old days, patients were examined in as much detail as my father, who was the chief of homicide prosecutions in Queens, investigated a murder.

So, let's skip the details on this patient, Peter Callas. Let's just say he was demented and couldn't remember from one minute to the next. He failed all the usual mental status tests. He had no idea who he was or where he was. He walked with the magnetic gait as described in Doctor Adam's paper. The nurses reported that Peter wet the bed, and he didn't seem to care he had wet the bed. His jaw hung, and he drooled. Didn't he realize it is not cool to piss in your pants or drool? He should be screaming, but he just sits there, staring blankly into space. What is he thinking? Probably nothing.

Lack of concern was also part of the more severe cases of the syndrome and was due to the tremendous dilation of the lateral ventricles of the brain pressing on and compromising the function of the frontal lobes of the brain. The lateral ventricles of the brain are some of the fluid-filled cavities in the center of the brain. Hydrocephalus is the condition where there is excess fluid in the cranial vault due to a defect in the normal resorption of the cerebrospinal fluid.

Conclusion: Peter Callas had the syndrome of normal pressure hydrocephalus. Now the question devolves into whether we can prove he has hydrocephalus and, more importantly, whether we can cure him of his affliction.

Each week, interesting cases from the ward service were presented to H. Houston Merritt, who was the chairman of the Department of Neurology at Columbia and at the same time the author of the foremost textbook of neurology at the time, and, at the same time, editor-in-chief of the *Archives of Neurology* (the foremost neurology journal of the time), and, at the same time, the dean of the medical school at the College of Physicians and Surgeons (the foremost medical school at the time), and, at the same time, vice president in charge of medical affairs of Columbia University (the foremost University...)—well, you get the picture.

That H. didn't bother me the way it bothered some people at Columbia-Presbyterian. It probably stood for Hiram or Henry or some other drab name Doctor Merritt didn't like. So, he called himself Houston. So what? He was a wonderful person, and a father to me and to the other residents. He had no children of his own, so he addressed us, his resident neurologists, as "his boys."

Merritt did have a dark side. He hated to lose at poker. Each month, "we boys" played poker with him at his home or the home of one of the other wealthy faculty members. We sat around a table drinking whiskey and smoking cigars like real men do and did in that era. If Houston was losing, his personality soured, and if he lost, if he had gotten behind the power curve, he took it personally and ended the evening angry at himself and, to a certain extent, at us for winning when he hadn't. Wisdom often comes in small doses. The wisdom of this experience for me was even great men can have their personal demons and foibles. But to his credit, Houston never had problems with temperament, problems that sometimes affect humans in their senior years. He was never full of himself, arrogant in his abilities, or condescending toward his subordinates. He always treated us, the youth, with a kind of great respect, almost reverence because he knew we were the future.

One of Houston's foibles was the side-splitting joke that he was fond of telling. I heard this several times from him as a medical student and twice as a resident:

"Jake stepped on a nail and got a puncture wound in his foot. He saw the doctor, who cleaned the wound and put on a bandage. A week later, Jake returned, and the doctor inspected the wound, cleaned it, and told Jake it was healing well. Jake shook his head and tried to speak, but only a mumble came out. The next week, Jake came with his teeth clenched together. The doctor inspected the wound and announced that it had healed. Jake couldn't speak, so he wrote a message: 'Do you think I have lockjaw?' The doctor looked Jake straight in the eye: 'Jake, why didn't you think of that sooner?'"

Houston's other big story was, "The Tomcat made too much noise at night, so they had it neutered. The next night it was out there making just as much noise. Now he, no longer a participant, was a consultant."

Another foible was reluctance to accept new ideas and new treatments, as illustrated by his opinion about my patient, Peter Callas.

H. Houston Merritt Makes Rounds in the First-floor Conference Room of the Neurological Institute of New York, 1967

Background Note: the Neurological Institute, affectionately known as Neuro, was founded in 1909. It was the first hospital in the United States dedicated to the care of patients with disorders of the nervous system. Though it has its own building and a distinctly separate identity, it is actually part of the Columbia-Presbyterian Medical Center. At Neuro, neurology and neurosurgery and neurorehabilitation are the only actions there are from the basement, where the neuroradiology staff works, to the top floor, where the neurological library is situated next to the office of the Head Neurologist.

Because Neuro is a teaching hospital, two things are going on at the same time— residents, fellows, and medical students are being trained, and patients are being taken care of. At Neuro, as was the case in all teaching hospitals in that era, the residents and fellows—collectively known as house staff—do and did most of the work and all of the heavy lifting. They are the doctors in training, and their fate is to get up early in the morning, work all day, and get to bed late at night or some nights not get to bed at all. Part of their job is to present interesting cases on rounds and conferences. What follows is a typical conference and presentation to H. Houston Merritt, the Head Neurologist at the Neurological Institute. The conference is taking place in the Zabriskie Auditorium, a small lecture hall on the ground floor. Two big doors with translucent glass panels and the words ZABRISKIE AUDITORIUM painted on them open on a room with a low stage on the south end. There are about 150 folding chairs that seat house staff and attending neurologists. The usual procedure is the patient waits while the history and the details of the case are reviewed for the group by the first-year resident neurologist, and then the senior neurologist in charge examines the patient and discusses what he thinks about the patient's problems.

Professor Rounds at Neurological Institute

Merritt: "History and CSF (cerebrospinal fluid)."

Me: "This 54-year-old has suffered progressive dementia over the last four years. He has become unable to feed himself, take care of his own toilet, and he is routinely incontinent of urine. His dementia has reached the point where he doesn't know his name and even where he is. He is totally dependent on others for care.

"The cerebrospinal fluid was under a pressure of 155 mm of water, clear, colorless, and had no cells and a normal protein and sugar. The test for syphilis was negative."

Houston Merritt then examines the patient and finds the abnormal gait, the complete dementia, and, yes, the patient had wet himself while sitting there in the wheelchair. The reflexes were hyperactive, and there were abnormal reflexes indicating dysfunction of the major motor tracts in the brain and spinal cord.

The Man Who Pissed in His Pants and Didn't Care

Merritt scratches his head.

"I don't know what is wrong with this man. The pattern of abnormalities doesn't fit with any known disease. He has more than Alzheimer's disease, and he does not have Parkinson's because there is no tremor or rigidity."

Merritt scratches his head, shakes his head, and eyes me suspiciously. He is truly puzzled and not happy he can't come up with a diagnosis.

"The best I can say is the patient might have multiple sclerosis. But with onset after age 50, and no exacerbations and remissions scattered in time and in the space of the nervous system, and dementia a major feature of this patient's illness, and a normal spinal fluid to boot—ugh! Multiple sclerosis is a long shot."

Ho ho ho. I have stumped the professor. That was the real goal of the presentation. My heart leaped for joy. This is the way progress is made. Youth tops the aged professor. New knowledge—it's delicious. And important. The hubris of youth propels us forward! The senior doctors have the money, but we have our youth!

Now I explain the Adams paper and what I am about to do to prove the patient has hydrocephalus. And that the correct diagnosis is normal pressure hydrocephalus, as discussed in the recent paper from Harvard.

"Doctor Merritt, I am going to put the patient in that special chair in the radiology department, and I am going to inject air into the spinal spaces and circulate air into the brain and the ventricles. I am going to outline the cortex of the brain and prove Mr. Peter Callas has no cortical atrophy, and, therefore, does not have Alzheimer's disease. Then I am going to expect that Mister Callas will quickly pass into coma because the air in the brain will further block resorption of the spinal fluid, decompensating a system already decompensated. The coma after pneumoencephalogram (our fancy name for the air in the spinal space procedure) is predicted by the Adams paper and, according to the paper, will support the diagnosis."

Note: these procedures sound primitive because they are primitive. It would be a mistake and an injustice to dismiss pneumography as some kind of medical freak show. This was an era before CAT scan, and the pneumo was the tool we had to use to visualize the brain. The whole procedure was going to be tough on the patient but important because we were doing something that had not been done before—initiating a new age in neurological medicine and surgery. We were going to cure a man of dementia.

I continued to address Doctor Merritt and the group of assembled physicians: "Jost Michelsen, my friend and ex-marine and ex-Harvard quarterback here, will be the neurosurgical resident helping me in this caper. Jost, take a bow." Jost waves. His face lights up like a kid's on his birthday. He shows his very large hands, the equipment he will use to place the shunt.

"Jost will be standing by to place in the dilated right lateral ventricle of the brain a low-pressure shunt whose opening pressure will be less than 155 mm of water. We then expect, and predict, Mr. Callas will awake from coma, walk and talk normally, and be restored to health."

Oh my God. To talk like that, I must have had a super gigantic ego. Looking back, I realize how ridiculous I must have sounded and looked. I never suffered with low self-esteem, not then, not ever. That is one of my problems, one of many personal defects.

OK. The conference is about to end. The great neurologist H. Houston Merritt now turns to Mister Peter Callas, the patient, my patient, and says, "The boys have terrible things planned for you. I advise you to sign out of the hospital as soon as you can."

There is more here than meets the eye. I was just beginning to find my way around the ego-clogged halls of big-time medicine. Ray Adams beat Merritt out for the chair of Neurology at Harvard. Thus, there is enmity, a good deal of enmity, between Houston Merritt and Ray Adams. Hence, Merritt does not believe in normal pressure hydrocephalus. Nor does Merritt believe in most of what Adams writes, says, or does. Socrates (Or was it Plato? Or both? Plato was Socrates' student and Socrates didn't write anything, so it must have been Plato who passed on the info or originated it.) pointed out, as I told you, the people who were most critical of cobblers in ancient Athens were other cobblers. The people who are most critical of neurologists are other neurologists. Who else would care? H. Houston Merritt's failing is a human failing and quite common in academic medicine. All of this was ironic because Houston died of low-pressure hydrocephalus. Before we get to that event, and the circumstances of Houston's death, let's get back to patient Peter Callas, who has just been told by one of the world's most famous neurologists to sign out of the hospital because "The boys have terrible things planned for you."

When he got back to the ward and his bed, patient Peter Callas had no memory of what Houston had advised, nor did he remember the conference centered around him and his case. His wife, who had attended the conference, said she trusted me more than she trusted "that old man downstairs."

The Man Who Pissed in His Pants and Didn't Care

"My husband is useless to himself and others. Try anything that might help."

The wife had what counts: the ability to exactly communicate the situation in a believable, human way.

So, with the wife's consent, we (Jost and I) moved forward with the treatment. Self-doubt had never been one of my strong points. Jost ditto. We knew early on; you sometimes have to do frightening and unpleasant things to patients. But, looking back on my behavior, I think by modern ethical standards, mine wasn't an acceptable, quiet kind of self-confidence. It was a brazen self-confidence, and I drew on it for this case and often lived on it. Was it justified? Who knows? Patient Callas needs help, really needs help. Don't you think? His disease is the problem, not me. For his sake and for the sake of science, why not follow the Harvard paper and see what happens? The alternative is to just let Callas vegetate in an existence hardly worthwhile or human. In his present state, he is useless to himself and a burden to others, particularly to his wife, who is the full-time caregiver when they are home.

Rapport Counts

The wife's ready compliance is one of the advantages of treating patients and family not as a stranger, but as a friend. In the old days, we called this close relationship between physician and patient good rapport. Rapport meant they would do almost anything asked. Good rapport meant the doctor always got permission for autopsy. I simply said, "We need to find out what went wrong so we can help others. Besides, it won't hurt. Dead bodies feel no pain."

In the old days, the patients and relatives were like Peter's wife. They thought we house physicians, the neurology residents, were their doctors, and they often stood up for us against the attending neurologists. The attending neurologists were officially in charge but limited their oversight to brief morning rounds. For the economically disadvantaged, the house staff was in complete command in the wards where these patients were admitted. Whoa! That reminds me of a side story that shows how a patient stood up for me. We'll get back to the Callas story soon.

Neurological Institute of New York
The Man with a Tumor of the Pituitary Gland

One time on rounds, I presented a patient to Doctor G. Milton Shy, another world-famous neurologist who had taken over as chairman of the Department of Neurology when Houston Merritt stepped down.

The patient had acromegaly from a pituitary tumor and was a giant of a big black man. Acromegaly is a disease caused by a small tumor in the pituitary gland, producing growth hormone. The patient's face slowly changes, becoming heavy and block-like with a massive jaw and forehead. The feet enlarge, and the hands become massive. The changes in my patient were especially severe.

His pituitary tumor had compressed the optic chiasm and was dimming the patient's vision, so decompression operation would be needed to prevent him from going blind.

On rounds, in front of my patient, out of the blue, Doctor G. Milton Shy asked me to name the 19 nuclei of the hypothalamus. I named three and could name no more. Then followed a tirade from Shy about how unworthy I was to take care of a patient when I didn't know the 19 nuclei of the hypothalamus. At that point, my patient turns to me and says, "Doctor Patten, who is this jerk? Should I beat the shit out of him?"

Me: "No, George, calm down."

George turns to Doctor Shy and addresses him directly: "I don't know who you are, buddy, but no one talks to my doctor like that. You betta get out of here before I belt you one." The big black man, my patient, then sits up and shakes his big black fist at Doctor Shy.

That'll teach Shy who is the real doctor around here. And that will teach him not to try to undermine the patient's trust in his doctor.

Shy made a fast retreat. He was guilty of pimping before medical residents, students, and interns had a word for his behavior. Pimping is the technique of trying to humiliate a lower ranked member of the medical team. Recent articles in the Journal of the American Medical Association discourage pimping because it does not have any proven educational value (ref: JAMA,314,22,2347-48).

Never Give an Irishman an Excuse for Vengeance

And vengeance came fast. I was not going to continue to work at Columbia when a jerk like Shy was chairman. That afternoon I called Doctor Fred Plum, the chairman of neurology at Cornell, and made arrangements with Fred to be his neurology resident at the New York Hospital Cornell Medical Center. At the end of the month, I would say goodbye to Shy by resigning my position at Columbia.

The Man Who Pissed in His Pants and Didn't Care

The next day, still at Columbia, we residents were making ward rounds when the overhead page announced, "Arrest, Neurological Institute Library." The top floor of the Neurological Institute had the neurological library and Shy's office. For some reason, the elevators were not working, so I and my fellow residents had to run up the stairs to get to the arrest scene. Let's see, that was probably from the fourth floor to the 14th. Maybe it took us eight minutes. While we were running up, I kept shouting and repeating, "This is great luck! Shy has arrested! We're rid of the son-of-a-bitch."

Imagine our surprise when we found Shy by the open window of his office unconscious. None of us made any effort to resuscitate him, for he looked dead. Instead, we just stood around with our arms folded. I volunteered to get the electrocardiograph machine. By the time I got back, Houston Merritt was there asking if we thought drugs had anything to do with this. Probably not. At yesterday's muscle biopsy conference, Shy told me, "It's not the present company, but I have a terrible pain in my abdomen."

Shy's autopsy showed a massive heart attack with infarction of the posterior inferior section of his heart. When the attack is there, in that location, the patient often does not have chest pain. They have pain in the, you guessed it, abdomen. Once again, I missed the diagnosis. But Doctor Shy missed the diagnosis also.

At autopsy, Doctor Shy also had a subdural hematoma compressing and displacing the right hemisphere of his brain, an injury we were told was left over from the war. People with right hemisphere dysfunction are often sons-of-bitches, and this may have been Shy's problem. If the right hemisphere is suppressed, the left takes over. The left hemisphere has its own agenda and often lacks feeling and rapport. That fact was demonstrated by Sperry's studies of humans who had their corpus callosum cut for the control of generalized seizures. In these patients, the left hemisphere takes charge of the right hand, and the right takes charge of the left. Arguments occur about what to wear. The right hemisphere goes for flashy colorful clothes and instructs the left hand accordingly, and the left hemisphere goes for more conservative apparel and instructs the right hand to pick accordingly. Sperry showed me a video of the right hand and the left battling it out over what to wear. The patient could not make up her mind because she actually had two minds in conflict. In another patient, the right hemisphere preferred a date with a go-go dancer. The left hemisphere favored a librarian. At one of the meetings of the American Academy of Neurology, I saw video where the patient was asked to tell about his motorcycle accident. The story came out with a great deal of emotion: "I was scared shitless, flying through the air, about to land and break my neck. Then I landed in some bushes that cushioned the blow. I was safe and sound. Thank God." Then a barbiturate was dripped into the right carotid to put the right hemisphere asleep. Now the story was told by the left hemisphere without prosody input from the right hemisphere. Now the story was flat, emotionless, and sounded robotic. "I hit a rock, tipped over, flew through the air and landed in the bushes." Same patient. Same event. But one was told with the shading and emotional resonance of the right hemisphere, and one was told with just the rigid and emotionless left hemisphere. These differences in hemisphere style and preference are quite real. You may have had the same experiences I have had at dinner parties. After a few drinks that have put the left hemisphere to rest, I hear myself telling the same story quite differently from what it sounded like when I was stone sober.

For demonstrating and documenting the hemispheric differences, Roger W. Sperry shared the 1981 Nobel Prize in Physiology or Medicine for "his discoveries concerning the functional specialization of the cerebral hemispheres." That year, the other half of the prize went jointly to David H. Hubel and Torsten N. Wiesel for equally important work on how the visual system processes information.

Whatever was Shy's problem, he learned his lesson the hard way: when you are not nice to your resident physicians, your resident physicians will not be nice to you.

Houston Merritt again became chairman of Neurology, and the gentlemanly ways of the Neurological Institute returned to normal. All was again right with the world. So, I called Fred Plum, told him what happened, and why I was staying at Columbia. Fred was irate. I don't blame him.

Back to Peter Callas, Normal Pressure Hydrocephalus, and Pneumography

Right after the air went into the spinal fluid space, we moved the chair around to outline the cortex of the brain. It was normal, as the Adams paper had predicted. The ventricles were not normal. They were massively enlarged, as predicted.

"Mister Callas, you OK?" I poked my head close to Peter's ear and shouted, "Mister Callas!"

No response! Callas was unconscious, as predicted. Now was time for Jost to do his thing and put in the shunt with a valve that would open at a pressure below the 155 mm pressure I had so carefully measured on the admission spinal tap.

The shunt, according to the Adams paper, would correct the hydrocephalus, decompress the ventricles, and restore the brain. For some reason, I was sure that would happen. Looking back on that adventure, I too am puzzled by how cocksure I was we would succeed. Was that the enthusiasm of youth? Yes and no. It was enthusiasm, alright, but I think it was an enthusiasm about science and the medical mission. Also, it took guts to try a new treatment. No guts, no glory. And the thing that made the whole thing possible was my rapport with Peter's wife. She knew I was taking care of them both as a friend and not as a stranger. Jost was part of the mission also. Without his full understanding and surgical skill, nothing good would have been possible. Jost was and is my kind of doctor: smart as the devil and, yet, a happy, pleasant person. His patients love him and for good reason.

Result

Anyway, I loved it. Sometimes it is necessary to be cocksure of something in order to make real medical progress. This was a chance to pull a demented person back to normal, a chance to recall Peter Callas to life. Think about that. How many times in a lifetime do you get a chance like that? A strange, foreign thought crossed my mind that it might be just as important to cure an individual patient of dementia, as it would be to make a great medical discovery. The reward of the patient's recovery now seemed almost as important as being a famous researcher, or having a high income, or making a substantial contribution to medical science. Helping people could be a goal in itself.

By the way, always bet on the reasonable, the probable, and the expected, as that is what is most likely to occur. That is your best protection against the unreasonable, unexpected, and improbable, and the unexpectable that may happen now and then. My bet was Ray Adams was right and what Adams said would happen would happen. How about you, dear reader? What's your bet?

Follow-Up

Within a week, Peter Callas was normal! Yes, normal. It looked like a miracle, and in a certain sense it was. It was a modern miracle based on the application of science at the bedside. Peter didn't remember much of the last four years of his life. He was like Rip Van Winkle learning what he had missed. His wife was overjoyed to get her husband back. Me too—I was overjoyed. I couldn't wait to present the patient and results to Doctor Merritt. I was sure that this one case was going to make a big splash. Why would anyone want to be president of the United States or the CEO of General Motors when they could experience the greatest joy of all by being a doctor who cured a patient of dementia? That was my thought at the time. Ah, medicine, nothing like it. Modern medicine is a more important invention than the internal combustion engine, and doctors are more important to humanity than the whole race of politicians put together.

H. Houston Merritt Makes Rounds in the
First-floor Conference Room

Merritt listened and then examined Peter. The mental status was normal, as was the patient's gait and station. The reflexes were also normal. So, what did the great man think?

Merritt: "This was placebo response in a suggestible patient. The shunt had nothing to do with this recovery. This kind of dramatic recovery only occurs in conversion reactions. All you proved was the patient was hysterical."

My jaw dropped. I couldn't say a word.

Peter Callas left the hospital a normal man. He stayed well for four months and six days when, unfortunately, he slipped while taking a shower, hit the side of his neck on the bathroom windowsill and broke the shunt in his neck under the skin.

The next day everything was back. He was demented, had the magnetic gait, and was incontinent of urine. His wife called, and I readmitted Peter to my service. What do you think was the problem?

Right! The shunt was broken and had to be replaced.

What should we do? How about repeat the pneumoencephalogram and prove the hydrocephalus had returned? How about just replacing the shunt? How about doing nothing and letting Peter stay demented, unable to walk, and incontinent?

I pause for reply.

What a wonderful opportunity to show the patient again to H. Houston Merritt and then redemonstrate the recovery.

Doctor Merritt again examines Peter. He found the patient completely demented, unable to walk, and incontinent of urine with obvious signs of organic nervous system disease (hyperreflexia, Babinski signs, etc.)

Merritt told the patient the same God damn thing: "The boys have terrible things planned for you. I advise you to sign out of the hospital as soon as you can."

Guess what the great man said when we represented Peter to him after the shunt revision? Right! Merritt claimed the patient had again responded to the operation the way a hysterical patient would respond to a placebo.

The Man Who Pissed in His Pants and Didn't Care

Coda: two years later, Merritt saw me in the hallway and grabbed me. "Thanks, Bernie, my boy, for the cigars you gave me for Christmas. I gave them to Mel Yahr. My doctor says I have claudication due to some obstructed arteries in both legs. The claudication is causing me to walk funny as if my feet were glued to the floor."

Subsequently, Merritt developed the triad of the syndrome of normal pressure hydrocephalus. The diagnosis was proven at the Neurological Institute of New York, but people at Neuro were reluctant to put a shunt in the great man. They sent him to Harvard, the Mecca for normal pressure hydrocephalus.

The irony: Merritt died in 1979 from normal pressure hydrocephalus, a syndrome whose existence he had never accepted during his career. The immediate cause of death at the Massachusetts General Hospital was an infection that complicated the neurosurgery that placed the shunt. Post-mortem examination of the brain showed significant vascular disease, especially near the surface of the ventricles. We now know loss of fine hair (ciliary) pump motion at the surface of the ventricle, due to vascular disease, delays the drainage of cerebrospinal fluid and can cause, in some patients, low pressure or normal pressure hydrocephalus.

Comment: one of my social dance students told me about her mother-in-law's dementia—dementia, magnetic gait, and incontinence. I told my student to get a neurological consultation. The internist on the case said the mother-in-law had Alzheimer's disease and a neurology consult was not needed.

Says I again, "Get a neurologist. The internist is wrong."

The neurologist said normal pressure hydrocephalus. The shunt restored the mother-in-law to normal mental functioning, stopped the incontinence, and produced normal walking. All that proved the internist wrong and the neurologist right.

My friend, an emeritus professor of radiology at the University of Texas Medical Branch in Galveston, started having trouble with unsteady gait and progressing to the inability to climb or descend stairs. His Mahjong game went down the tubes, and so did his memory. He says he never developed incontinence of urine, but his wife says he wet the bed. Anyway, it turns out any part of the syndrome may be absent in some cases. My friend responded to a lumbar shunt and regained his excellent memory and skills at Mahjong. His magnetic gait disappeared, but he still needs a cane because of vascular problems in his legs. My friend, too, like Peter Callas, had trauma that broke the shunt. The syndrome returned and then disappeared again when a new shunt was placed.

My take on the situation is that normal pressure hydrocephalus is lots more common than people imagine. A 2007 survey of several nursing homes and chronic care facilities turned up normal pressure hydrocephalus in 9% to 14% of the inmates (inmates? —a Freudian slip, I mean residents) in those institutions. Reference: Marmarou, Anthony, Young, Harold F, Aygok, Gunes A; Estimated incidence of normal pressure hydrocephalus and shunt outcome in patients residing in assisted living and extended care facilities. Neurosurgical FOCUS 22 (4) 1-8, April 1, 2007.

Lesson: It would be a good idea to find, diagnose, and treat these people who have normal pressure hydrocephalus. Many are probably in nursing homes, wasting their lives and waiting for death.

Talking about the pneumoencephalogram in Peter Callas reminded me of the pneumoencephalogram almost done on a special patient of Doctor Michael E. De-Bakey, the world-renowned cardiac surgeon and my boss at the Baylor College of Medicine. Here's the story of how and why a horse was admitted to the Methodist Hospital.

Tableau Twenty-One:

A True Horse Story

Methodist Hospital, Houston—Now Known as Houston Methodist

Leon Jaworski called Doctor DeBakey about Leon's horse stumbling around the pasture. Could something be done to help?

And yes, friends and readers, this is the Leon Jaworski who founded the international law firm Fulbright & Jaworski. The same Leon Jaworski who headed the investigations into Nazi war crimes that led to the Nuremberg trials and the very same special prosecutor who toppled Richard Nixon, forcing Nixon to release the tapes that showed Nixon knew about the Watergate break-in. Leon is his nickname. His full name is Leonidas, after the Spartan King who is remembered for his heroic death at the battle of Thermopylae. Leon has a brother named Hannibal, in case you didn't know. So, someone in the family knew history or had a sense of humor or both.

A Horse is Admitted to the Hospital

Doctor DeBakey admitted Leon Jaworski's horse to the Methodist Hospital for diagnosis and treatment. Yes, you read right. The horse was admitted to the hospital.

Two neurologists were called in to consult on the horse's problem. One of those neurologists was Ben Cooper (who is dead), and the other does not want his name connected with the events about to be narrated. So, I will call Ben Cooper BC and call the other neurologist, who wants to remain nameless, AC.

The horse was under anesthesia in the radiology suite on the second floor on the east end of the hospital. When the neurologists saw the horse, it was lying on its right side and was fast asleep, due to the deep anesthesia.

BC: "Ataxia in this fine animal. Too bad. Probable cerebellar tumor. Don't you think?" That's the way Ben Cooper talked, "fine animal" is classic Ben Cooper talk. But I can't duplicate here in print his accent, which was South African. Nor can I show his smile, which was a smirk.

AC: "Yep."

BC: "If this fine animal has a cerebellar tumor, removing fluid from below might cause the tumor to shift and compress the brainstem. That would end things for this fine animal and begin quite a lot of not-so-fine trouble for us."

AC: "No diagnosis. No treatment. No pneumo. No diagnosis. How about we do a cisternogram?"

Note: AC is suggesting putting the needle in the spinal fluid at the level of the cisterna magna (neck region) instead of down below in the lumbar region. Air can be injected into the cistern and the cerebellum outlined that way. Cisternal puncture might be safer if the horse had a cerebellar tumor. Thank God we don't do pneumoencephalograms anymore. The scans give much better pictures of the brain, much faster, and with much greater safety. But this was the old days, and we had to work with the tools we had.

BC: "Have you ever done a cisternogram?"

AC: "On humans, yes. On a horse, no. But it has to be similar. Just stick the needle in the cistern and pump in the air."

BC: "Right. Right. Right. Check the fundus. Make sure this fine animal has no pap."

Note: as explained in The Engineer with the Subdural Hematoma, pap is an abbreviation for papilledema, a swelling of the optic nerve in the back of the eye that would indicate the pressure in the brain is elevated. If the pressure in the brain were high, the danger of the spinal tap would be greater than if the pressure were not elevated. So, Ben, who always had the take-charge attitude and was a control freak before we had the term control freak to describe such people, was telling AC what to do to see if the horse had evidence of increased intracranial pressure.

AC struggles to get the horse in better position and then announces, "Can't see a blessed thing. The media is clouded."

BC: "Give me that ophthalmoscope, you-son-of-a-bitch. Your generation doesn't know how to do much of anything."

Ben now tries to see into the back of the horse's eye. "God damn. This fine animal has bilateral cataracts. They are opaque and yellow. That is a hypermature cataract. Has some special name. I forgot what."

AC: "Morgagnian cataract. That's the name in humans. About horses, who knows? But bingo! That's the Dx (Dx = diagnosis). The horse is stumbling because it can't see."

David Patton, the chairman of the Department of Ophthalmology, while the horse was still under general anesthesia, then removed the cataracts. David probably also placed plastic lenses in there to help the horse see. I am not sure exactly what David did. I wasn't there when he did it.

Leon was happy, and so was the horse. The horse returned to normal and no longer stumbled in the pasture.

MED—Michael E. DeBakey

In those days, Michael E. DeBakey was enormously powerful. If he wanted a horse admitted to the Methodist Hospital, then that is what happened. Here is an example of Doctor DeBakey "requesting" a consultation. Doctor DeBakey went by his initials MED, with the E standing for Ellis, his middle name.

Doctor DeBakey "Requests" a Consultation

My family and I were having a nice late-night dinner at Café Annie, one of the great restaurants of Houston and the world. It was 10:30 p.m. when the great man called.

MED: "Doctor Patten, this is Doctor DeBakey."

Me: "Yes, Doctor DeBakey, I recognize your voice."

MED: "Doctor Patten, Oscar Wyatt's cook had a seizure or something that caused her to fall off her stool and fall unconscious on the kitchen floor. I want you to do a consultation on her tonight and have a note in the chart by 6 a.m. tomorrow morning when I make rounds."

Me: "It's pretty late. Can't it wait until morning?"

MED: "No. This is Oscar Wyatt's cook. Make sure your note is on the chart by 6 a.m."

Note: Oscar Wyatt is a multimillionaire oilman and has a reputation for making big donations to worthy causes.

Ethel and Craig stayed in the car while Allegra, my daughter, and I consulted on the case of Oscar Wyatt's cook. I don't recall what time it was, but I am sure it was after midnight when Allegra and I got to the patient's room, which was on the fourth floor of the main Methodist Hospital.

The patient was a big black woman, a big black mama, who tipped the scales at 682 pounds. She needed two beds to contain her bulk, and there was a special lift at the bedside the nurses used to turn the woman, who otherwise would have been difficult to move, if not unmovable. As a cook for one of the wealthiest men in the world, this patient probably had eaten many fine dinners. Too many.

She was asleep but snoring loudly. The snores would increase in loudness, and then they stopped altogether. When the snoring stopped, the patient became restless, seemed to awake partially, clutched her throat, and grunted. She had stopped breathing for one minute and 47 seconds by my watch, and then, with a loud sucking noise, fell back asleep and started snoring again.

My note: this patient has sleep apnea due to upper airway obstruction. She fell asleep on the stool in the kitchen and fell to the floor. A sleep study will confirm the diagnosis. Signed, Bernard M. Patten.

At 6:25 a.m., I am awakened by Doctor DeBakey.

MED: "Doctor Patten, this is Doctor DeBakey."

Me: "Yes, Doctor DeBakey, I recognize your voice."

MED: "Doctor Patten, I read your consultation note. It is short and to the point. I like that. But you better be right."

Comment: the sleep study confirmed the bedside diagnosis. The patient started weight reduction and had an operation to open the upper airway. Sleep apnea is a type of sleep disorder, as was shown in this patient. Usually, there are pauses in breathing during sleep that can last up to several minutes and may occur many times per hour. When the breathing stops, as it did in this patient, CO_2 builds up in the blood, and the brain wakes the patient to start breathing again. The breathing lowers the CO_2 and increases blood oxygen, and the patient falls back to sleep. The diagnosis is made by observation at the bedside, as it was in this case, and confirmed by a sleep study, which is also called a polysomnogram. Most cases of this condition are due to upper airway obstruction, as was the case here. Some cases are due to a defect in the central nervous system, and some are due to obstruction and a defect in the central nervous system. All the cases that I saw in my practice were obstructive or obstructive and central and were accompanied by very loud snoring. All the cases that I have seen have had excessive daytime sleepiness, which interfered with safe driving. Symptoms can be present and undiagnosed for years. The key thing to remember is that a negative sleep test does not rule out the diagnosis. CPAP (Continuous Positive Airway Pressure, invented by Colin Sullivan in 1981) is a great treatment for the sleep apnea syndrome and has obviated, in most cases, the need for surgery.

While we are on the subject, I want to tell you more about MED.

Soon after I came to Baylor, I was making rounds with the resident and spotted an old man who looked like he had fallen asleep waiting for an elevator. "Go help that old guy. He fell asleep while standing up," said I.

"That's Doctor DeBakey," said the resident. And it was. Legend has it, Michael Ellis DeBakey, known in the Texas Medical Center as MED, got only three hours of sleep a night so he could have more waking hours to be productive. Whether true or not, I don't know, but I do know MED usually looked like he needed a good night's sleep, and he sure looked like he was asleep the first time I saw him.

What else can I tell you about MED?

MED's favorite poem was Thomas Gray's "Elegy Written in a Country Churchyard" (1750). His favorite part of the poem was lines 33–36:

The boast of heraldry, the pomp of pow'r

All that beauty, all that wealth e'er gave

Awaits alike the inevitable hour:

The paths of glory lead but to the grave.

My take on this is MED believed that, in the end, no matter what … we are still human and only that. No matter what we have or have not, we still will die. But I also think that MED believed good deeds and what we and he accomplish live on to help others.

MED sometimes recited Gray's cheerful lines at faculty meetings. They reflected his fatalistic philosophy and not his Maronite Catholic religion. My father liked to start the day by holding up his glass of orange juice and saying, "Another day and another step closer to the grave." That was typical Irish fatalism and has nothing to do with my father's Roman Catholic religion. I like to think my father was warning us to use our time wisely, and I like to think MED was doing the same.

> **Lesson:** Time is precious. Use it wisely.

MED did have a dark side, which I hesitate to talk about. He fired William Fields, who was the chairman of Neurology at Baylor who hired me. Fields' job was taken over by John Stirling Meyer, who was subsequently also fired by MED. The reason these great neurologists lost their positions is not clear. MED had a blind spot about neurology. MED often said, "If you can't cut on it, or cut it out, what good is it?" meaning that surgery was the only effective treatment of anything. I personally agreed with MED. In that era, the really scientific part of medical practice was surgery. Internal medicine was mainly bluff and conjecture, and neurology was a branch of internal medicine, the foremost branch, I might add, because at least we knew the anatomy of the nervous system, a knowledge based on basic science with great diagnostic accuracy but very little therapeutic effect. At least the surgeons could do some good by either "cutting on it or cutting it out."

But you know, usually there is a stated reason for things, and there is the real reason, which is not stated. About the reason Fields got the ax, I know nothing. John Meyer did tell me how he was fired by MED. Meyer was called into MED's office. There was a yellow envelope on the desk. MED pointed to it and told Meyer to pick it up. The letter said, "Because you have failed to develop adequate programs in neurology, you are relieved of your responsibilities as chairman."

Meyer had a personality similar to MED and probably, for that reason, antithetical to that of MED. Meyer (and Fields) had serious questions about the reported benefits of carotid surgery, as performed by MED. Meyer also was a world's expert in measuring cerebral blood flow. There is speculation the cerebral blood flow measurements before and after surgery showed no benefit from the surgery. It is a fact that, after Meyer was fired, he was forbidden to do any cerebral blood flow measurements at Methodist Hospital. It is also a fact that Meyer moved his entire research laboratory to the Houston VA Hospital where he continued his National Institutes of Health supported research in cerebral blood flow. Meyer had tenure as a professor and, therefore, could not be fired as a professor. He could be demoted as chairman, but his position and salary were guaranteed by tenure.

MED was the only physician at Methodist Hospital permitted to maintain his own records. Therefore, it was not possible to check MED's reported surgical results against the actual patient records. Henry McIntosh, the chairman of the Department of Medicine, left Baylor about the same time that Meyer was fired. Henry went to work at a Florida health organization, and David Patton left Baylor to enter private practice of ophthalmology at a hospital in Flushing, Queens. Baylor politics was a lot more serious than democratic politics in Queens. And at Baylor, the fighting seemed to be over trivia. For instance:

Fighting over the Size of Erections

After MED fired John Meyer, Robert Williams, the chief of psychiatry, was appointed acting chairman of Neurology. He appointed me vice-chair, and it fell on my shoulders to do the administrative work of the department. That was one big pain in the ass. There were lots of meetings I had to attend, and in each meeting, I felt I was bleeding. Faculty members bugged me for everything under the sun: more space, higher salaries, more people to help them, more resident coverage of their private patients, parking closer to the medical school, and so forth. These supposed adults were crying whining babies. And I had to run the residency program and also the clinical practices committee. On top of the problems handling these babies on the neurology faculty, there was the problem of the Neurosensory Center of Houston.

John Stirling Meyer had gotten the money together to construct a center for Neurology and Neurosurgery, similar to the centers that existed in other medical centers and similar to the Neurological Institute at the Columbia-Presbyterian Hospital in New York City. The first snag was that the neurosurgeons were unhappy about their participation in the building. They were to have one-third of the space, and they were to pay for it. For some reason, I think lack of money, they backed out. That problem solved itself when the Department of Otolaryngology (ENT) stepped in to take the place of the neurosurgeons. So, to this day, the neurosensory center has three divisions: Eye on the south side, Neurology in the middle, and ENT on the north. Neurosurgery is not a part of the neurosensory center.

The next problem was more daunting: MED sent out letters saying all construction for the neurosensory center must stop. MED claimed there was not enough money to proceed with the project, but I knew that was not true. Besides, even if it were true, we could always count on the rich people of Houston to come to our aid.

It was Robert Williams, the chief of psychiatry, who figured out what the real problem was. He also suggested the solution citing an analogy: "The Baptists have to have a higher steeple than the Methodists."

Me: "I don't get it. What do church steeples have to do with hospital construction, Bob?"

"Lots! We are dealing with a primitive male concern about the size of erections."

"You're joking."

"Nope. The problem is the neurosensory center was to be taller than the cardiovascular building. Therefore, the problem was that Meyer's erection, the neurology building, was to be bigger than DeBakey's erection, the cardiovascular building. This, of course, sounds absurd. It sounds absurd because it is absurd. But if my psychoanalytic appraisal were true, then the solution would be to sign papers promising the plans for the neurosensory building would change, and the neuro building would never exceed the cardiovascular building in height."

And so, following the psychiatric advice, I promised Doctor DeBakey in writing that the neurosensory center would never be taller than his heart building. That is, I promised that neuro's erection would always be less than cardio's erection. Men fighting over the size of their erections—it was cliché, but, in this case, it seemed real.

It Was Real

Bingo! MED agreed to let construction continue, and that is why there is a Neurosensory Center of Houston.

Tableau Twenty-Two:

The Marvelous Effect of Placebos

Baylor College of Medicine

Neurology residents at Baylor put on a show each year at Christmas time. One of the skits was always about Doctor Patten treating over one-third of his patients with placebo. That was a gross exaggeration. The percentage was more like five, and those patients were happy and also experienced few side effects. Alas, the era of placebos is over for ethical reasons I don't understand. Here's how the placebo worked in the good old days of yore.

Blue Placebo Was the Most Powerful

Methodist Hospital had three placebos: red, white, and blue. If one did not work, you could switch the patient to another. In my experience, the blue worked the best. For example:

A 10-year-old boy was referred for evaluation and treatment of his muscle weakness, which had progressed over a five-year period to the point he couldn't walk. So, he made his way around in a wheelchair.

On examination, he was weak with small muscles in no particular distribution. The muscle biopsy showed non-specific abnormalities, which consisted of small muscle fibers of both type I and type II. The type I fibers are the slow oxidative fibers, and the type II are the fast glycolytic fibers. Multiple blood tests were normal, and the electromyogram showed features typical of muscle disease, something we knew already. The kid had a muscle disease. But what was the cause? The muscle enzymes in the blood were normal, so the muscle itself was not breaking down. In short, after a pretty exhaustive investigation, there still was no explanation of the weakness. There was no diagnosis. No diagnosis was the end condition of about a third of the patients I took care of. These days, techniques and tests are more effective, and I would estimate only about 10% of patients end up without a definite diagnosis or without a clear explanation of the cause of the problem.

So, what do you do if you don't have a diagnosis? What do you do if you don't know what to do? Answer: analyze the situation and act accordingly.

The parents and kid were told I could not come up with a specific diagnosis, but I would like to try a treatment.

"The treatment is very powerful, and we will have to watch for side effects. Start with three blue capsules a day and call me in two weeks to report on how you like the treatment and how the treatment likes you."

Mom called the next day: "It is too powerful for him. He is shaking all over and feels too much energy."

Me: "Wow! That is a very good sign. Let's cut the dose and build up slowly over several weeks until he can tolerate the full dose."

Over the next six weeks, the dose was increased by one capsule every two weeks. The results speak for themselves. The kid got out of the wheelchair and walked. Eventually, he returned to normal and was able to play basketball at school. All this occurred because of the blue placebo, which consisted of small amounts of a three-carbon sugar called lactose.

The following year, there was a convention in Houston of the medical directors of the muscular dystrophy clinics of Texas. They asked me to discuss the diagnosis and treatment of the kid, who had been followed in a muscular dystrophy clinic for the duration of his illness. In particular, the doctors wanted to know how I cured the disease and what the effective treatment was.

They were told about the work-up and the lack of a specific diagnosis. Then I asked the family to leave the room. I told the doctors about the blue placebo and how I had touted it as a powerful treatment, which, in this case, it was. With but little understanding of the disease process, I had, by prescribing, a completely inert substance, caused my patient to improve, recover, and prosper. I was brimming with pride. My placebo treatment had outdistanced all of the latest discoveries in the medical journals and textbooks. I had cured my patient using airy nothing!

Woe is me! I had thought I was in for excellent accolades for curing this kid with absolutely nothing but faith in a placebo. I was wrong. Just the opposite was true. The reaction was extremely unpleasant. The clinic directors thought I was a charlatan, a faker, a quack, and they derided me and the treatment. But, of course, they had a hard time explaining the result. They did have the good sense not to inform the parents and the kid, for that may have broken the spell. My own conscience is clear because I regard the practice of medicine as a kind of sacred calling (like that of the ancient priests, medicine men, shamans, and sorcerers), in which we are to use all the means at our disposal, even magic, even airy nothing to help the sick, and I believe we are to do it with close personal relations with the patients and, as Morton Thomson advised, NOT AS A STRANGER!

The good result continued. When the kid applied to law school, the school was concerned the illness might recur. My strong letter stating a recurrence was unlikely, and I thought the disease had disappeared for good helped the law school accept him. He is now the District Attorney of one of our esteemed counties in Texas.

This patient taught me a great lesson. The quacks and the fakers probably helped many of the suckers who paid them for snake oil. The snake oil salesman is either a charlatan or a healer or both, depending on the circumstances and the results. The same relations apply in alternative medicine: expectation of the patient and belief in the healer. Physical therapy, occupational therapy (both of which I prescribed often) and acupuncture—ditto.

Medicine is an art, a science, and (God help us) a business. The use of placebo was part of the ancient art of medicine. Scientific studies show conclusively placebo is often effective. That is why the prospective, controlled studies of treatments, and new agents and operations now require that part of the study include a measure of the placebo effect. One of the interesting results of such studies was the finding that a significant number of patients taking only placebo have significant side effects! The shaking and surge of energy that the kid experienced while taking three blue placebos a day is a startling example of side effects from placebo, which are now officially called Nocebo effects.

The other way to use placebo is by intravenous injection. That can be effective in the conversion hysterias when all else fails. For example, there was a woman with paralysis of both legs. She did not like the kind of probing needed to get to the intrapsychic conflict that was causing the problem. I had to use something else. That something else was strong suggestion in the form of an intravenous injection of normal saline (saltwater balanced to resemble the osmotic strength of blood). This treatment is most effective when accompanied by a drama at the bedside. So, I would announce to my entourage of medical students and residents and nurses, that I was going to try a new powerful treatment, "Desperate situations require desperate treatments."

Then, I would tell the head nurse: "Prepare my special treatment, the intravenous injection."

The nurse would bring a 50cc. syringe (a big one!) filled with saline and hand it to me.

Then I would explain to the group: "This treatment is so powerful and so effective, I alone have to give it and will not let a mere resident or intern give the injection."

And then, with a flourish, I would slowly inject the saline into the patient's arm vein while she is lying there in bed looking like a wilted flower.

Bingo!

"Doctor Patten," she says. "My legs are tingling!"

"Good! That's the beginning."

"Oh my God! My legs are twitching. Look at them. They're beginning to move."

And then, in front of the medical students, nurses, student nurses, interns, and residents, this previously paralyzed patient, with a flourish, swings her legs around, plants them on the floor, and gets out of bed and walks! Another cure as dramatic as any described in the Holy Bible!

Her husband was grateful for my restoring his wife to health. For many years thereafter, he was a big supporter of my research. Neither the husband nor the patient ever asked what was in the injection I had given at the bedside. If they had asked, of course, I would have told them, "It was a medicine, a powerful medicine!"

Logic: yes, where is logic? Where is it, for instance, in the next moment of this story? Dante said, "To appreciate the good, we need to discuss things that are not so good." And that is what I am about to do. Here follows one of the worst mistakes I ever made. If I had the chance again, I would correct it. Even now, I can't imagine how I could have been so stupid.

Tableau Twenty-Three:
Mistakes Were Made

Baylor College of Medicine

The patient was in his fifties and had a minor genetic muscle disease for which he was getting some symptomatic treatment. If this sounds vague, it is because it is vague, deliberately so because his medical condition doesn't concern us here.

He worked for a gigantic chemical plant in Beaumont, Texas as the environmental protection officer in charge of certifying vats of chemicals for burning at night. The routine, as he told me, was to do a chemical analysis of the liquid in the vat, and if it was safe to burn, seal it with his certification it contained no prohibited substances.

It rained one night after he left the plant. He decided to go back to get his umbrella. Then and there he saw something strange. A truck pulled up to a vat he had certified. The driver opened the seal and dumped something in the vat. The vat was then resealed, and the truck left.

Retest of the vat showed PCBs had been added. PCB (perchlorinated biphenyls) may cause autoimmune disease and do cause cancers in animals. PCBs were banned in the United States in 1974 and banned by the Stockholm Convention on Persistent Organic Pollutants. As usual, there are exceptions to the ban, including closed systems as in hydraulic fluids and transformers where the PCB supposedly cannot find its way into the environment. It is illegal to burn or discharge PCB into the night air except under special conditions of hyperoxygenation and high-temperature ignition (1,200 degrees or higher). Burning PCB under those conditions is prohibitively expensive. Burning PCB under routine conditions produces extremely toxic dibenzodioxins and dibenzofurans. Further nighttime snooping revealed the company routinely added forbidden materials to the certified vats and burned them. Over the course of about seven months, my patient kept a careful log of all the details of the crime—time, place, truck number, materials added, and so forth. Damning evidence.

In clinic, he told me, "Congratulate me. I am about to blow the whistle on the company and the people involved. This will be the most important thing I will ever do in my life. Monday, I will go to the federal EPA (Environmental Protection Agency) and tell them all I know."

I was elated and told him he was a great hero protecting the public health from the polluters who would damage the public health for their own profit.

This is my reading of what happened then. Or rather, this is my reading now, of my reading of what happened then and why it happened. The son of a District Attorney should have seen what was coming, should have warned about what can happen, should have advised the patient to make multiple copies of the evidence and distribute it many places. I should have told him to make sure the people he talked to knew there were many copies of the evidence and his friends were to blow the whistle in the event anything should happen to him. I was swept up too much in this man's enthusiasm and forgot about the problems associated with real criminals and real crime. I had stopped thinking and was celebrating the downfall of the wicked we thought was about to happen.

Two weeks later, I got a call from the Greek Orthodox priest in Beaumont.

Priest: "The family said I should talk to you. They say this was not a suicide. They say he was murdered."

Me: "What? What are you talking about?"

Priest: "He didn't answer his phone. The relatives went to his apartment. They found him dead, hung on his own shower head with the shower water still running."

I told the priest the story.

Priest: "He will be buried in sacred ground."

That was an ordinary sad story—all too familiar—and simply told. Does character develop over time? In novels, it does. But in real life? I am ashamed that I, who had heard at the dinner table about murderers and murders, about real BAD Guys in the old days of my youth, had failed to foresee this murder. Shame on me.

Let's pause to praise famous whistleblowers. There is free speech in America, but you have to pay a price for it. In 1777, Samuel Shaw and Richard Marven witnessed their commanding officer torture British prisoners. When they reported this to the Congress, they were arrested and jailed. The following year, Congress passed a law protecting whistleblowers, and Shaw and Marven were acquitted by a jury. My personal hero is Frank Serpico, who exposed corruption in the New York Police Department. Frank suffered. During a drug raid, he was shot in the face. Fellow officers did not call a 10-13 (officer shot). An old man in the apartment called 911 and stayed with Frank, who was bleeding.

At the Knapp Commission (appointed by Mayor John V. Lindsay) Frank famously said, "police corruption cannot exist unless tolerated at the highest levels in the department." He was awarded the medal of honor, the highest honor. He says there was no ceremony. The badge was just passed across the desk like a pack of cigarettes.

Then there is the famous case of Karen Silkwood who worked at Kerr-McGee Cimarron Fuel Fabrication near Crescent, Oklahoma. She made plutonium pellets for nuclear rods and she mysteriously was contaminated with plutonium several times. On the way to talk with David Burnham (New York Times), her car crashed, and she was killed. The pack of documents carried on the front seat of the car was never found. The rear of her car had been hit by another car, and that may have pushed her car off the road. Blood levels of lutes were high, so she may have just fallen asleep at the wheel. Subsequent investigations showed contamination of her home and her boyfriend's and 44-66 pounds of plutonium missing from the plant. The plant was decommissioned, of course.

Erin Brockovich exposed Pacific Gas and Electric for contamination of water with hexavalent chromium. Sharon Watkins exposed accounting fraud at Enron. National Security Agency contractor Edward Snowden leaked classified information about illegal wiretapping of Americans. These are heroes who seek truth and justice even in the face of great personal risk.

Praise them.

> **Lesson:** Yes, it is still happening today. One must be very careful when blowing the whistle. Ugh! Cover your ass. CYA is good advice.

There follows another patient whose problems I could have handled better. The next mistake had national and international implications.

National Institutes of Health
Dmitri Dmitriyevich Shostakovich—Russian Composer
Background

In 1973, Dmitri Dmitriyevich Shostakovich came to the United States seeking a diagnosis and treatment for his chronically progressive nervous system disease that had caused weakness and atrophy of his right hand. The medical visit was sponsored by the U.S. State Department and the Soviet Union under the condition that the great composer would make no direct statements unless they had been filtered through and approved by the Soviet agents who came with him.

Due to the complexity of his medical problems, Shostakovich (nicknamed "Mitya") was admitted to the medical neurology service at the Clinical Center of the National Institutes of Health in Bethesda, Maryland.

On admission, I found him to be a sad, bitter, decrepit, depressed man who was shy, nervous, and awkward. His distress was magnified by the constant presence of his Soviet handlers and the fear he might say or do something wrong. He obviously thought it was absurd he was not permitted to answer my questions, even the most banal medical questions, without the question first being posed to the KGB person in his room. The KGB person would then say the question to Mitya, who replied in Russian, and then the KGB person would tell me the response. This led to more than the usual delays in getting a medical history and doing a complete physical and neurological exam. It was annoying not to be in direct contact with my patient. Getting a good history is the key to understanding disease and often predicts the future. And in getting the history, the patient's tone, body language, and so forth are important in evaluating the situation.

"Why can't I talk with him directly?"

"That was not in the State Department agreement that conditioned his coming here."

"The American State Department agreed to prevent a patient talking directly to his physician. How come?"

"Shostakovich's English is so poor what he might say or what he might not say may be misconstrued."

"OK. I'm fluent in French. How about I talk to him in French?"

"His French is so poor he might say or might not say something that would be misconstrued."

"You're good, a really good translator. Most Americans wouldn't know what misconstrued meant."

"Thank you, doctor."

"This is bullshit. I don't believe this great composer, Mitya, a known polymath, doesn't know French or, for that matter, English."

The KGB man says nothing—just shrugs his shoulders and smiles. He holds his hands out in the position of a suppliant to indicate "What can I do."

Lesson: Soviet oppression was real. Direct censorship of even great artists was the rule, despite the enormous waste of time and energy involved.

Shostakovich's Medical Problems

My patient was in chronically poor health. He suffered from severe emphysema, probably caused by the Russian cigarettes (the name of which I can't recall) he chain-smoked daily. His heart was moderately diseased with residual damage from the heart attacks in 1966 and 1971. Chest x-rays showed old inactive lymphatic tuberculosis, which he had contracted in the Spring of 1923, but there was no evidence of the lung cancer that would kill him in 1975, two years after he left the Clinical Center at Bethesda. From trivial falls, the patient had suffered two broken legs (right and left). His bones were demineralized, probably from poor nutrition in his youth (he had practically nothing to eat during his stay at the Petrograd conservatory). Excessive smoking and possibly some genetically controlled metabolic bone disease contributed to the weak bones. His cervical spine was short, stiff, and had limited ranges of motion in all directions. There was tenderness over the fifth, sixth, and seventh cervical vertebrae. There was a history of injuries to the neck from falls. He was extremely nearsighted with the usual retinal changes of extreme myopia. Because of poor eyesight, he was rejected when he volunteered for service against the Nazi invasion of Russia on June 22, 1941.

Shostakovich's Neurological Problems

The patient said he did not know when his hand started to get weak, but it must have been before 1959. By 1966, even before the heart attack, the patient was unable to play the piano in concert due to right-hand weakness. The atrophy and weakness had been diagnosed in Moscow as "chronic polio," a disease not recognized in America at that time or any time—a disease which the Soviet physicians made up to explain the weakness. Chronic polio does not exist. Polio is an acute viral illness, never chronic. There has never been a case of polio lasting 14 years (1959 to 1973). The diagnosis of chronic polio may have been a way that Soviet physicians kept their true diagnosis from Shostakovich. It may have been their name for chronic progressive spinal muscle atrophy, a type of motor neuron disease, which is usually fatal.

The neurological examination showed that the patient had a severe spinal cord compression at the seventh cervical level, with increased reflexes and spasticity below that level. The right hand was atrophic and useless. Sensory changes were present in the distribution of cervical roots five, six, and seven, more on the right than left. From the examination, it was clear that Soviet physicians had not known the true nature of their patient's illness and that it was potentially treatable.

Lesson: Soviet medicine was poor. The ignorance of Soviet physicians was vast. Any qualified neurologist should have been able, from examination, to determine that the patient had a compression of his cervical spinal cord from a subluxation of the cervical vertebrae, such that the bony parts of the neck were compressing the spinal cord and the nerves in the neck producing the sensory loss and weakness detected on examination.

Shostakovich's Psychological and Psychiatric Status

My patient had problems all right. None psychiatric. He has had no hallucinations, delusions, or illusions. His reality testing was normal. True, he appeared nervous and had multiple tics. But he had none of the known neuroses. Instead, he had realistic reasons to be afraid. Stalin had been in power. Now the equally bad Brezhnev had taken over. The Soviet government was increasingly repressive; artistic works were judged by the standards of Soviet ideology. Anything modern or dissonant was denounced as "formalistic." Formalistic music was a serious offense against revolution, against the people, and against the state. The definition seemed to be anything that sounded modern was formalistic and, therefore, bad. But in reality, it was anything that seemed to offend the communist party.

For example, The Nose (Shostakovich's first opera) was slammed by party critics. The next opera, Lady Macbeth of Mtsensk, provoked charges of writing "modernistic bourgeois" music and (the more serious charge) the crime of "musical formalism." This came from Stalin himself who, after act one of the opera, stomped out of the theater, livid and enraged over what he called "that degenerate music." The following day, Stalin dictated an article for Pravda entitled "Muddle or Music." The next day, January 28, 1936, the article appeared in print. It shocked the Soviet musicians and the musical world by denigrating the opera. Even more ominous, the article ended with an undisguised threat, a threat from Stalin himself who had unlimited power and was used to using that power and, on many occasions, used that power in the most disgusting, hideous ways. In those days, if I had Stalin as an enemy, I would live in fear. You would too. So, in my view, Shostakovich's nervousness was justified by the grim objective reality in which he had to live.

Recall that Stalin was searching for scapegoats for the failures of his five-year plans. Accusations of sabotage, espionage, wrecking, musical formalism, capitalistic sympathies, anti-proletarian ideas, hoarding, etc. etc., became convenient methods for both transferring blame and eliminating political opponents by show trials, death squads, exile to Siberia, long prison terms at hard labor, etc. etc. etc. Thus, the universal climate of fear, distrust, and suspicion that characterized the Stalinist era and the era that followed Stalin that Shostakovich was forced to deal with.

Not only was Stalin against him. The Central Committee of the Communist Party released a resolution (March 1948) that all musical works should have a socialist content. Then, believe it or not, the party closed the Soviet Union to all Western music. The music of Schonberg, most of Stravinsky, Hindemith, Bartok, and Weber (I am not making this up) was banned. Music was to be evaluated only on the basis of "doctrinal purity." Sergey Prokofiev and Shostakovich were singled out for their "unhealthy individualism and artistic pessimism" and their "spirit of negative criticism, despair, and non-belief."

Tikhon Khrennikov, appointed by Stalin to administer Soviet music, attacked Shostakovich at the first Composers' Congress:

"Armed with clear Party directives, we will put a final end to any manifestations of anti-people formalism and decadence, no matter what defensive colouration (sic) they may take on." The Congress unanimously condemned "formalists" Shostakovich, Prokofiev, Khachaturian, and other leading composers.

According to R.J. Rummel (*Lethal Politics: Soviet Genocide and Mass Murder Since 1917*), Stalin and the Soviet government were responsible for 61,911,000 nonmilitary deaths. By contrast, Hitler and the Nazis were responsible for 20,949,000 nonmilitary deaths, roughly one-third the Soviet number.

These figures on Soviet deaths are not "Red Scare" numbers prepared by McCarthyite propagandists. If anything, the information now coming out of the former USSR shows the estimates are too low. In his book *Testimony*, Shostakovich said, "You have no idea what it's like to live in a totalitarian state. To tell a joke to a friend, you must go to the bathroom, run the water full force, whisper the joke into your friend's ear, and then laugh in cupped hands. [To survive] It was not enough to love Soviet power. Soviet power had to love you."

He should know; Shostakovich was purged twice, in 1936 and in 1948. Then he was rehabilitated twice. Then he was denounced again for his usual big sin: formalism.

His works were periodically banned. When he was fired from his teaching job, he had to play the piano at silent movies to make a living. What a waste!

On several occasions (probably with a gun to his head), he had to apologize to the public and to Stalin, and regrettably, denounce fellow musicians who were imprisoned or executed. He wrote a symphony (no. 13 called Babi Yar) that acknowledged the Holocaust at a time when official Russia did not. Consequently, his family's privileges and his own were withdrawn. According to Professor Greenberg (cf. notes), one punishment was cutting the water off at the Shostakovich family's apartment. At other times, Shostakovich kowtowed to the politburo and the Kremlin, toed the Party line, and publicly said what he was told. Much of this duplicity, necessary for survival, caused guilt and self-loathing—the secret inspirations (I believe) behind much of his music.

On my orders, the nurses paged me when the KGB agents left for the night. Without them, Shostakovich was a new person—friendly, happy, funny, and interesting. The nervousness and the tics were no longer in evidence.

The story he told that I liked the best, the one we both laughed at, and the one that shows much of his private character as opposed to the public mask, was the story of his studentship at the Leningrad Conservatory:

"One day, I was informed I would be required to pass an oral exam in Marxist ideology. About this subject, I knew little."

Convinced that he would fail, he joked about his "pianistic reliability versus his political reliability."

The exam was given December 1926 and was administered by a commission. The question was, "explain the differences, from sociological and economic standpoints, between the work of Chopin and Liszt."

Shostakovich broke into hysterical laughter so strong that it would not, could not stop. He was dismissed from the exam without having answered a single question. Instead of answering a question, he had doubled up laughing his head off and was carried out of the room.

In my view, this question is so emblematic of the stupidity of Party hacks that when I heard it, I rolled off my chair laughing just as Shostakovich did.

Laboratory Results

The myelogram confirmed some spinal cord compression with impingement of nerve roots as they exit the spinal cord. The cervical subluxation was considered significant by radiologists.

Treatment

I suggested surgery to stabilize the cervical vertebrae, to try to stop the progressive weakness by decompression of the spinal cord and to give a chance for recovery of function.

Follow-up

Soviet leaders, Brezhnev included, doubted that their doctors could have been so wrong. They asked me to consult others to confirm or deny my diagnosis. So, I asked for a consultation by Doctor Daniel B. Drachman, a professor at Johns Hopkins. Dan felt that we should have additional consultation from the chairman of his Department of Neurology, so he brought Doctor Guy McKhann along to help. After detailed review of the data, repeated examinations, much soul-searching, and, I believe, calls to other people around the country, the two consultants gave it for their opinion that the cervical spine should be decompressed.

Dan: "You know, Bernie, you are playing with fire."

Me: "Yes, so what?"

Dan: "If something goes wrong, the Soviets will blame you and America for damaging their national hero."

Me: "Humm."

Dan: "Send him back to Moscow with a strongly worded letter giving the recommendation that surgery be done there. That gets him out of our hair and us off the hook."

Me: "Guy too? Does he agree?"

Dan: "He agrees on the need for surgery. He has no opinion about where or when. That's up to you."

The State Department agreed sending him back seemed prudent, but I should do whatever I thought was best. There was never a question of money, as the United States National Institutes of Health had agreed to pay for any and all medical expenses. And there was never a question of who would make the final decisions about the treatment and surgery. I was the doctor, and I had to do the deciding.

Lesson: I made a mistake. Without personally knowing the medical situation in Russia, I should not have sent Shostakovich home for surgery. From what I personally observed about the KGB and their brutal management and control of this great musician, I should have realized what would happen.

Back home, Shostakovich was again told his condition was due to "Chronic Polio." In a letter to me, Soviet physicians informed me they now agreed that there was spinal cord compression due to the subluxation, but they thought the spinal cord compression was an incidental finding and the real cause of the problem was "Chronic Polio." They added that even if the spinal compression was causing the problem, such an operation could not be done in the Soviet Union. On this point, they were right. Later on, in 1986, when I visited the Soviet Union, I saw that Soviet medicine was at least 40 years behind the times, and that Soviet ignorance greater than I had ever imagined. The misinformation, propaganda, politically managed science had taken its vast toll. Not only did Soviet doctors not know much, much of what they thought they knew was actually wrong! They believed their own nonsense; they believed their own bullshit. The Soviet physicians I met and talked with believed they were infallibly right, as they believed the forces of history were infallibly on their side. They had a complete and utter lack of understanding of neurology and of science as we know it. The Soviet Union had excelled at producing tanks and rockets but failed miserably at producing decent health care. They had impressive-sounding research institutions and thousands of professors, most of whom were appointed for political reasons and not merit. The reality was their doctors were poorly trained, and their hospitals were terrible, no better than what one might find in the worst third-world country. Believe it or not: the main hospital in Moscow had its entire supply of medicines for the whole hospital stored in a two-by-two-foot glass case! Anything you could name was in short supply, including penicillin.

Shostakovich Expressed His Disappointment with Me
and with Dan and Guy

"My American doctors ...bragged that they would cure me without question, they had made such great progress in the field, and so forth. And now all they talk about is courage."

Dmitri Shostakovich, Testimony, page 214 (reference below).

> **Lesson:** VIPs sometimes get lousy medical care.

> **Lesson:** Politically managed medicine and politically managed science = disaster.

Closing quote from the man himself:

"No, I can't go on describing my unhappy life, and I'm sure that no one can doubt now that it is unhappy. There were no particularly happy moments in my life, no great joys. It was grey and dull, and it makes me sad to think about it. It saddens me to admit it, but it's the truth, the unhappy truth."

Dmitri Shostakovich, Testimony, page 214.

Subsequent Course

The weakness and disability continued to progress. Shostakovich became an invalid, then bedridden. He died on August 9, 1975 of cancer of the lung. A civil funeral followed. The body is interred in Novodevichy cemetery in Moscow.

The obituary was signed by Brezhnev, who called Shostakovich "the greatest composer of our time" and a "hero of the Soviet people."

Peroration and Conclusion

If Shostakovich were here with us, I think, he would say he was no hero. In the Soviet Union, heroes died young. By 1953, the year Stalin died, there were few anti-Stalinists above ground. Nope! Shostakovich was a survivor, not a hero. His music is a testament to what he saw and felt in a world so grim none of us can imagine what it was like to be him.

Coda

I called the record room of the National Institutes of Health Clinical Center, the hospital where I had taken care of Shostakovich for over two weeks. They told me they have no records about Shostakovich, and they have no record of his admission to the clinical center. Then I called Dan Drachman at Johns Hopkins and asked him to fish out his record of his consultation. The next day, Dan called back. "The file is gone. We have no record of my ever having seen him. Our records department can't explain this, and neither can I. Guy's records are gone too."

I sent Dan this narrative of what I remember about the case. Dan said that is the way he remembers it. "The cervical spine and nerve roots were impinged, and he needed surgery."

Conclusion

It is hard to believe that Soviet agents removed records from the Clinical Center and from Johns Hopkins Hospital. The records must have been removed by agents of the American government acting under authorization from the State Department.

Some references for those interested:

- Teaching Company, Chantilly, Virginia, 2002.

- Shostakovich, Dmitri, and Volkov, Solomon, *Testimony: The Memoirs of Dmitri Shostakovich*. Harper and Row, New York, 1979.

- Wilson, Elizabeth. *Shostakovich: A Life Remembered*. Princeton University Press, Princeton, 1994.

- Conquest, Robert. *The Harvest of Sorrow: Soviet Collectivization and the Terror-Famine*. W.W. Norton, 2001.

- Figes, Orlando. *A People's Tragedy: The Russian Revolution, 1891-1924*. Penguin, 1998.

Lesson: Russia is a different country. Different countries are different and do things differently.

Lesson: The political system of a country counts and sometimes counts a lot.

Baylor College of Medicine
More Mistakes—Death Related to Informed Consent

Changes in ethics have altered the patterns of medical practice and medical research in America. The full impact of changes in ethics is not known, and probably will not be known for some time. Any change in ethics should be subject to the same strict scientific standards that apply to any other aspect of medicine. There should be double-blind prospective controlled studies to see if ethical rule Y + X gets better, worse, or the same results as Y. Until we see the results of detailed, unbiased studies, demonstrating favorable risk-benefit ratios, cost-effectiveness, and lack of significant adverse effects, we should not conclude that any new ethical rules (usually made ad hoc by some bureaucrat in an office somewhere far, far away from the laboratory or the clinic) are necessary, needed, or beneficial. On the contrary, wisdom dictates that customs long established should not be changed for light and transient causes. Some physicians have pointed out adverse effects of new rules. Ingelfinger, one of the great physicians of all time, pointed out in *Annals of Internal Medicine*, 83;264-269, 1975, the unethical nature of some of the newer medical ethics. He was concerned, as are we all, with the alarming trend toward the dilution and depreciation of the important by a proliferation of the trivial. I know that physicians reading this will know exactly what I am talking about.

Too Much Trivia is the Current Problem and a Major Concern

Some patients will also know because they have found their doctors are so busy typing into the medical record that they don't seem to pay attention to them or even look their way. I had a lawyer who treated me that way. Dropped him like a hot potato. I had a dermatologist who treated me that way. Dropped her too.

Patients and physicians deluged with consents and releases may lose sight of and respect for the important issues. For instance, the 1975 Office for Protection from Research Risks Rule requiring informed consent to retain for research purposes an organ or fragment thereof removed at autopsy—even when done in accord with reasonable and customary medical practice—has no basis in law or supports in the courts; yet, it still remains a requirement and continues to waste the time, energy, and money of one of America's scarcer resources, the trained clinical investigator.

Let's face it: medicine and medical research are overregulated. Their mission to serve humanity is encumbered by the large number of regulations now governing them.

Informed Consent

Somewhere, sometime, a lawyer had an idea that the case he/she was handling would go better in court if a stricter standard were applied to the consent. Consent to an operation would not be good enough. It would have to be "informed" consent, and the informed part would be pretty open-ended on how much risk need be discussed and consented to. When something went wrong, as it may, then the issue might be raised that the consent was not informed and that it was merely consent and not informed consent. Thus, the pressure is on to discuss with patients a lot more of the potential risks, even though the probabilities are miniscule. Not only is the cost of medical care increased because physicians spend more time explaining the obvious and not-so-obvious medical risks, but also there is danger that complete information may generate uncontrollable fear or irrational rejection of a needed treatment.

Just before I retired, the consent forms the patients were required to sign ran several complicated pages. None of my patients ever read them. They just signed. I never read them either. Think of all the time I have saved by not reading these bullshit forms.

My feeling is that the following two patients suffered from attempts to obtain informed consent. I obviously did not do well by patient one. Patient two was lost because his doctors didn't like him, and they made the informed consent the excuse to make the patient refuse treatment.

Baylor College of Medicine
The Welder

A 52-year-old welder was in excellent health until involved in an automobile accident. Following the accident, he developed pain in his back and severe pain in the bottom of his right foot. Multiple treatments, including bed board, heating pads, pain pills, and muscle relaxants gave no relief of the foot pain, but the back pain did improve a great deal. He had been a welder for more than 17 years and was proud of his skill and his earnings, which were $17,000 a year. That year (1973), my Baylor salary was $35,000, and I had earned $7,000 more from my private practice. Me too. I was proud of my take, for it was much greater than I had ever earned in a year by working. I mention his obsession with his work because his main concern, expressed to me many times, was to get back to work as soon as possible. I didn't blame him. For a high school drop out to earn that kind of money in Texas at the time was amazing.

Neurological examination showed weakness of the extensors of the right big toe, decreased ankle reflex on that side, and decreased pin sensation on the bottom of the right foot. X-ray showed he had six instead of the normal five lumbar vertebrae. The myelogram showed impingements on the nerve roots at lumbar 5-6 and lumbar 4-5. The impingements looked trivial and probably did not explain his foot pain.

What did explain his foot pain was the electrical studies of his nerves. He had tarsal tunnel compression of the right tibial nerve. The distal latency was 8.2 milliseconds. Bingo! We had a diagnosis and a very treatable condition. The nerve was entrapped by a connective tissue scar. The scar was caused by the trauma to the foot during the accident. All that was needed to stop the pain was to release the nerve by cutting the band of fibrous scar tissue that was compressing the nerve. This was going to be another great cure!

The day before the scheduled operation, the neurosurgeon tried to get informed consent, truly informed consent, by telling the patient that the operation might cause hemorrhage, infection, paralysis, or death. All of that was true of course, but very unlikely because all that was needed to release the compression was a simple incision under local anesthesia.

The patient signed himself out of the hospital.

At home, according to his wife, the pain continued. He told his wife that there wasn't much for him to live for because he could not work, couldn't stand the pain, and the surgeon told him that there was a possibility that the operation might result in paralysis or death.

One day, when the pain was particularly severe, he went to his backyard, put the muzzle of his shotgun in his mouth, and pulled the trigger.

Three days later, his letter to me arrived at my home. It read, "I decided not to have the operation because Doctor XXXX----- told me it was very dangerous and couldn't promise me if (sic) it would be successful and said there was always a chance of being paralyszed (sic). The pain is too much. I have no reason to live."

The neurosurgeon on this case a few months before had a million-dollar judgment entered against him for the malpractice of his resident. The neurosurgeon's earnest desire to comply with legal requirements in order to avoid further litigation probably explains his vivid description of the possible consequences of surgery, which, after all, was only the release of the tarsal tunnel under local anesthesia.

My patient, a man with no medical experience, was not a great intellectual. There was no reason that he should be. Great intellectuals make poor welders and vice versa. He was no intellectual, but he was not stupid. Fundamentally, he was a sincere, simple man who would have been better served by rather limited information about what might happen. It is a pity that the patient interpreted the explanation of possible complications to mean the surgeon did not want to do the operation and did not believe it would help the pain. That led the patient to think there was no hope for his condition. Extinction of hope, according to Beck, is the single most important factor leading to suicide. The depression caused by the illness, the pain, the lack of income, along with the seeming hopelessness of the situation, probably led to the patient's suicide. Thus, this patient did not benefit from attempts to get his informed consent. On the contrary, there was an adverse effect of that attempt that was as serious as the most serious side effect that could have happened from the operation.

Sometimes I wish clinical medicine were more like chemistry where everything is predictable. But it isn't and never will be because medicine deals with humans. Humans are much more complex than any chemical. Good fiction writers know they have to show characters that exhibit enough conflict and contradiction so that we can recognize them as belonging to the contradictory human race. Nonfiction writers do not have such need. They just have to show people as they are—exhibiting conflict and contradictions every goddamn day.

I should have talked to the patient before and after the surgeon to neutralize the poisonous effect of complete informed consent. Or even better, I should have done the operation myself in my office under local anesthesia. It would have taken a few minutes, and Dale, my operating room nurse, could have set things up and assisted me.

Here's the consent I should have asked the patient to give: "The nerve in your foot is compressed from a scar that formed after the accident. The electrical test shows compression at an area of the nerve no wider than the tip of a pencil. I will go in there under local anesthesia and cut the band of tissue compressing the nerve. The whole operation will last less than five minutes, and I expect that will relieve the pain right away. OK? If you agree, sign here."

Now in retrospect, I realize I should have done the release of the nerve myself and not consulted a neurosurgeon. After the experience with this patient, I did all the peripheral nerve operations and biopsies myself. In general, that worked out, except one patient sued me for malpractice. Her story will come up soon.

Mistakes Were Made

Informed Consent Hurts Another Patient

A 54-year-old lawyer developed severe substernal crushing pain that increased with exercise and decreased with rest or nitroglycerin. Because the chest pain worsened over a three-month period, and the nitro had less and less effect, angiocardiograms were done. They showed segmental occlusion of two coronary arteries. A bypass operation was proposed. In view of the patient's occupation, complete disclosure of risks and possible benefits of surgery were reviewed with the patient over a two-hour conference, filmed for the record. After the conference, the patient refused surgery. One month later, this lawyer suffered a heart attack and died on the way to the hospital.

This lawyer's health adventure had an insistent appointment-in-Samarra aspect. If he had been an ordinary citizen and not a malpractice lawyer who had successfully sued many local physicians, I think the minutiae of cardiac surgery and anesthesia would not have been explained as extensively in an attempt to get informed consent. And, sad to say, from a realistic point of view, it is probable the doctors didn't want to have anything to do with this guy, and I don't blame them. Maimonides said, "Make friends with your physician before you get sick." That is good advice. In this case, the physicians erred by deliberate over-disclosure of surgical risks so that the patient would reject the procedure, which might have saved his life. If the surgeons had given this lawyer the usual discussion of risks, he would have accepted them and accepted the operation the way most patients do. By the way, the surgeons involved in the lawyer's case had developed this operation to a high art. They did 17 to 20 such operations a week, usually without much trouble and usually without complications. Those surgeons can do that operation in their sleep. So, they should not have made it seem like such a big deal. It wasn't.

References:

Holder AR, Levine RJ; Informed consent for research on specimens obtained at autopsy or surgery: a case study in the overprotection of human subjects. Clin Res 24:68-77,1976.

Beck AT, Kovacs M, Weissmann A: Hopelessness and suicidal behavior. JAMA 234:1146-1149,1975.

> **Lesson:** Sometimes, less informed consent is better than more. Why make a mountain out of a molehill? Why kill a chicken with a cow knife? Tailor the consents to the individual patient's needs.

215

Baylor College of Medicine
Another Mistake—I Fail to Make a Correct Diagnosis

He was a 29-year-old petroleum geologist with a Ph.D. He did lots of field work doing seismographic analysis to discover oil deposits. In the field, he slept in a tent and, on multiple occasions, he was bitten many times by deer ticks. About six months prior to the time he came to clinic, he noted he was getting tired easily. Subsequently, he had trouble with walking over uneven ground and stumbled and fell several times. Eventually, he developed foot drops and weakness of his arms and legs. There was no rash, no fever, no swollen joints or lymph nodes. About two weeks prior to his office visit, he noticed trouble swallowing and weakness of both sides of his face. His neurologist in Tyler, Texas, thought George had motor neuron disease and sent him to me for a second opinion.

General physical examination was normal. Neurologically, he was weak with grips of 18 pounds (normal for age is better than 86). Upper and lower extremity muscles were small, and he had to use two Canada crutches to walk. Sensory testing was normal to pin, vibration, soft touch, and position sense.

Ugh! It looked like he had a motor problem alright, and it was either in the neurons or in the axons or in the peripheral nerve.

All the blood tests for the usual collection of autoimmune diseases were normal. The nerve conduction times were normal, but needle electromyogram showed denervation. Muscle biopsy had lots of neurogenic degeneration of both Type I and Type II muscle fibers. No inflammation was seen. The nerve biopsy showed degeneration of myelinated and unmyelinated fibers and loss of axons. Small patches of chronic inflammation with lymphocytes were present. The spinal tap, in my view, was the most revealing. Spinal fluid was completely normal except for three oligoclonal bands. Oligoclonal bands indicate antibodies are being produced within the nervous system. This is abnormal and indicates an immune reaction to something. The interpretation I gave it is that George had an autoimmune disease of the nervous systems. I guessed that he was producing antibodies against his nerves, and those antibodies were the cause of the nerve disease that produced his severe weakness. If that guess were true, he might respond to immune suppression treatment.

Not knowing what to do, I decided to sit on his case a while and do some library work for more information and do some thinking. Meanwhile, George stayed in the hospital.

Mistakes Were Made

Three days later, waiting for me in my office was Amber, the night nurse on Jones nine, the neurology service at the Methodist Hospital.

"Amber, what the hell is wrong. You look terrible."

"Doctor Patten, I am terrible. I did a terrible thing last night. I will resign my position at Methodist and seek psychiatric care."

"Would you like some tea or a cappuccino? I have a machine here to entertain the students and residents, but nurses can drink coffee too."

Amber shakes her head no and slumps down on my office blue leather couch.

"You know that geologist patient?"

"George?'

"Yes, George. Last night he looked so miserable when I made my rounds, I decided to cheer him up by giving him sex. I know it was unprofessional in the extreme. Sorry."

"You had sexual intercourse with George in his room in the hospital?"

"Yes. Last night, about 2 a.m." Amber bows her head and wipes her eyes.

"How was it?"

"Very weak. He's very weak. Lots of trouble getting it up, but I finally got him up with my mouth. I had to get on top and pump and pump and pump, but I finally got him off."

"Do you want my advice?"

"I already decided to report myself to the nursing board. They will take away my license. I know that. Is that what you're driving at?'

"No, Amber. Are you kidding! You are not a good nurse. You're a great nurse. Stay on the job. Just forget it. And don't tell anyone what happened. Go thy way and sin no more."

"You're quoting Jesus from the Bible."

I nodded and smiled. Jesus often gave excellent advice.

Hell, Amber was just helping my patient by being compassionate. It sounded like the sex was consensual.

What would you do, dear reader? Report Amber, or let it slide?

Amber continued on the job, and George continued to go downhill.

Every Thursday, I made rounds by myself. Other days, I am surrounded by interns and medical students, so Thursday is my chance to talk to the patients directly and find out what makes them tick. This was face time before that term had been invented. That evening, I made rounds on George.

"Doctor Patten, the nursing service here is super. I especially want to commend Amber for her excellent service. She is so sweet and so caring and so kind and so wonderful."

"I'll let her know."

Result

Steroid treatment didn't work. George went downhill. He refused respirator care and died at home. There was no autopsy.

Ten years later, at 2:35 in the morning, I woke up in a cold sweat. In my dream, I realized George had Lyme disease. He should have been treated with antibiotics. I completely blew the diagnosis, and that is why George descended into dusty death.

Lyme disease, caused by a bacterium, Borrelia burgdorferi, and spread by deer tick, can result in serious nervous system disease like the one George had. The other possibility was tick-born Ehrlichiosis. But George didn't have flu-like symptoms that usually go with that condition, and there was no fever or chills usually seen in Ehrlichiosis. Lyme disease it was, and I missed it. The oligoclonal bands in George's spinal fluid were probably directed against the Lyme agent. On the other hand, some patients with Lyme also develop autoimmunity and require dual treatment: one treatment against the infection and one treatment against the infection-induced autoimmunity.

Ugh! I also missed the even bigger picture that George did have a motor neuron disease and that a motor neuron disease could be caused by an infectious agent. My thinking was too conventional, too narrow. George, with his signs and symptoms and downhill course, could easily have been sold as a motor neuron disease sufferer. Henceforth, because of George's case, I shall force myself to start thinking in ways that are counterintuitive. Such reasoning is generally wrong but sometimes can result in a major breakthrough. For instance:

Is There an Infectious Cause of Motor Neuron Disease?

Come to think on it, I have consulted on and done muscle and nerve biopsies on patients with AIDS who looked, for all the world, like they had Amyotrophic Lateral Sclerosis (ALS). Yet, those patients with antiviral treatment stabilized, and some even recovered from AIDS and ALS. Could some cases of ALS actually be due to an infectious agent? Behind closed doors, we muscle experts wondered why some of our colleagues who specialized in the care of ALS patients came down with ALS. That could have been a coincidence, of course, but I doubt it because ALS is a rare disease, and I think too many ALS specialists have died of the disease.

The Texas Nursing Board Would Have Removed Amber's License

Personally, I don't think what Amber did is right, but I don't think making a big deal about it is right either. Making small things into a big deal is a fundamental modern problem, not just in medicine, but with our society in general. Let me cite some examples:

Example 1: a child died in a swimming pool in Houston. So, the mayor and city council of my little village, the City of Taylor Lake Village, decided to consider passing an ordinance that required every swimming pool in the village to be enclosed by a wire fence, so that children could not easily enter the pool area without adult supervision. My arguments against that were:

1.   The pool in Houston was fenced, yet the child died anyway because mom left the area to go to the bathroom. Therefore, adult supervision is better than a fence. Why not make it a law that in a pool area, adults must supervise children who can't swim?

2.   If we really want to prevent death from pools, we should drain all the pools and fill them with cement. That would prevent any deaths from pools and eliminate any need for a fence.

3.   As our fair city is surrounded by lakes (Mud Lake and Clear Lake and Taylor Lake), the lakes also should be surrounded by wire fences because the water in the lakes can cause death from drowning just as easily as water in a pool.

Result: no ordinance. No pool deaths in 40+ years. Conclusion: pool fences are not needed in our community. But overreaction and political hysteria tried to push us in that (wrong) direction.

Example 2: there is a park south of our home on Baronridge Drive. A man wrote the city council that he was concerned about the safety of his four-year-old daughter who had to cross Baronridge to get to the park. He wanted a stop sign put on Baronridge to make cars stop. He thought that would prevent deaths from kids getting hit by cars as they tried to cross Baronridge to get to the park. My argument against the stop sign was:

•   Stop signs may not solve the problem because cars may not stop. What we really need to prevent accidents is a policeman stationed at the crossing 24/7. Whenever a kid wanted to cross, the cop would escort them.

Result: the city put up a stop sign. The Texas Department of Public Safety made the city take it down. It turns out you need to do a traffic survey for two years to determine if a stop sign is really necessary. Such a survey must be paid for by Taylor Lake Village government and would cost about $40,000.

Result: so far, over two decades, there have been no injuries or accidents involving kids crossing the street. The four-year-old in question made it to the park safely many times. She is now 27 years old and married with three children of her own.

Example 3: the bridge over Armand Bayou was lowered to prevent boat traffic from entering Mud Lake and heading north to Armand Bayou Nature Center. Bill Fisher, the former astronaut, Marta Greytok, our mayor, and I went to Austin to ask for a change order.

Sidebar: Bill is one of the smartest persons I have ever known. He and I had a great discussion of American history on the airplane up to Austin. His knowledge of American history is encyclopedic. When we got to the airport, Bill bought a hot dog and probably put too much mustard on it. When he squeezed the bun, the dog slipped out and fell onto the airport floor. Bill picked it right up and shoved it in his mouth, saying that he had eaten much worse in space. I'll bet he did.

Marta's arguments slip my memory. Bill was full of facts and maps. His main point was that with heavy rains the present bridge would impede the flow of water from the Bayou into Clear Lake. That would increase the chance that homes along Armand Bayou, his home and mine, would flood. My arguments were two in nature: a girl had been decapitated while trying to water ski under the lower hanging bridge nearby. She, evidently, thought she could make it, but a wave or something elevated her just as she went under the bridge, and that was that. My other argument was, "In medicine when we make a mistake, we get busy and correct it right away. This bridge is a mistake, so let's correct it." That argument begged the question, of course, and I didn't expect much effect. Begging the question is an error in argument because it assumes something is true when that something is actually under examination. Here, I stated that the bridge is a mistake. That statement begged the question by asserting what I was supposed to prove. On the other hand, the art of rhetoric is to select from the available materials the arguments most likely to be effective. Often, making a bullshit assertion the way I did is more effective than proving things by facts, figures, and maps. The art of rhetoric also teaches the most effective arguments are those that are emotionally, not rationally, based. Indeed, the argument that worked in this context took place after the formal hearing.

The new commissioner came out to the lobby. He said, "Wow! You, sir, are an extremely effective public speaker. Where did you learn to speak like that?" His question was never answered. Instead, I used my psychiatry training to advantage.

"Commissioner, I understand you are new, just appointed. Here's your chance to show these engineering types who's the boss. Just order the change."

Two days later, he called me and told me he had ordered the change, and it would cost the state $125,000.

Result: the bridge over Armand Bayou does not impede the flow of water into Clear Lake. Over a 10-year period, I saw no boat traffic headed anywhere near Armand Bayou Nature Center. Each year, I sent a letter to that effect to remind people what they thought might be a problem was no problem at all. They never replied. They never admitted they were wrong. To expect some people to admit a mistake is to expect too much.

Tableau Twenty-Four:

Patients Predict Their Own Death

Brookhaven National Laboratory, Medical Research Center, 1963
Patient Beatrice

The first patient who did that was a patient of George Cotzias at the medical research center at Brookhaven National Laboratory. She was a wonderful person with lots of endearing features, including a sense of humor and an uncanny ability to imitate George Cotzias.

Beatrice, a patient with lupus, had him down pat, even the Greek accent and the way Cotzias would explode: "Bureaucrats! They seem to think that the only way to advance is by obstruction. They talk an idea to death. The guys who run this place are the world's foremost experts at squashing good ideas. That's because unimaginative people like them have one absolute favorite use for their formidable intelligence: telling other people, especially people with formidable imaginations like me, with total conviction and logic, why new ideas won't work."

"This afternoon I will die," announced Beatrice Weaver during morning rounds.

"Death, hey! Too bad we can't help with that, but if there is something else, we can help with, tell us," said Cotzias, flashing that affected grin of his.

"I have a headache," said Beatrice while clutching her forehead.

Cotzias ordered a Darvon.

Nurse Petersen, as prim and proper as ever, poured a glass of water and gave it to Beatrice. She placed the Darvon in the patient's outstretched palm and stood back.

Beatrice glanced around the room. She took a sip of water and slowly moved her right hand toward her open mouth. Just as she was about to pop the red and blue capsule, Cotzias shouted, "Stop!" The room reverberated with the roar of his voice.

Beatrice arrested her hand in midair, just in front of and to the right side of her opened mouth. She looked at Cotzias expecting another order, but instead, she got a question.

"How's your headache?" he asked.

A surprised look appeared on the patient's face. She hesitated and, looking at the ceiling as if for inspiration, replied, "It's gone."

"Thank you for that wonderful demonstration!" said Cotzias as he turned and left the room.

Beatrice followed him out. She still held the Darvon in her right hand in front of her face but at chin level. "What should I do with the Darvon? I don't need it anymore," she asked.

"Take it anyway," sneered Cotzias.

Cotzias turned to me and, while Beatrice stood next to us, said, "She feels deprived of tender loving care. She just wants us to do something for her. We're giving the others attention, which she craves, so she has to butt us to get some attention for herself. Mel, please check her. Bernie, you help. Try to find out why she will die this afternoon. If possible, do something to prevent her death."

I followed Mel and Beatrice back into her room.

Mel tried to clarify the situation by asking questions. She insisted she felt fine but knew, nonetheless, that she was going to die.

Mel listened to her heart and turned the stethoscope over to me. I heard the normal lub-dub. Mel thumped her back and listened to her lungs. They were normal, too. He felt the abdomen, liver, spleen, kidneys—all normal. He checked reflexes and had the patient walk about. Normal results again. Mel shook his head. He licked his lower lip and ordered a chest x-ray and a bunch of blood tests.

"Beatrice, you seem OK," he said. "We'll just check a few things to make sure."

"Doctor Van Woert," said Beatrice, "I am OK. It's only that I am about to die. Before I die, I want you to know how much I appreciate the excellent care you and Doctor Patten and all the doctors gave me. And after I'm gone, I don't want you to feel the least bit responsible for my death."

She was hysterical. I hoped Mel would tell her off. Instead, Van Woert replied, "Thank you. We do our best."

Mel and I went to the doctors' conference room to await the blood tests results. As soon as Mel sat down, he got up again and ran back to Beatrice's room with the EKG machine.

I helped hook up the leads while Mel read the tracing: "Normal sinus rhythm, normal rate at 76, normal P, QRS, Q-T interval, and T wave. All that shows the atria, and the ventricles are normal. Let's go look at the chest x-ray."

The chest x-ray was normal, too, as were the blood tests, including complete blood count, serum potassium, sodium, glucose, calcium, phosphorus, bicarbonate, chloride, blood urea nitrogen, blood oxygen and carbon dioxide—all normal. Everything Mel could think of was normal.

Beatrice looked just as she always had. The tests were all normal, yet Mel kept at it.

"Mel, I don't get it. We examined her. We did the tests. Everything is OK. So why worry? Just tell her off. She's hysterical, seeking attention, the way Cotzias said. And wasting our precious time."

Mel shook his head, exhaled a sigh, and explained. "God, I wish medicine were that easy. If it were, a technician with a cookbook could do it. But it isn't. I've had cases like this before. The patient senses something wrong. The doctors don't know what it is. That's a bad combination. Confusion in the mind of the physician is the single most important bad prognostic sign. And I am confused. Under the existing state of the art, that's where we stand. I can't think of anything else to do. Can you?"

"Sure, I can. Go in there and tell her off. Tell her that she is a crock of shit. Tell her she has wasted several hours of our precious time. Tell her that we can't give her MSH or any of that other stuff because she doesn't have Parkinson's disease. Next week, or the week after, or sometime, we may get around to trying an experimental treatment for lupus on her. Meanwhile, she must be patient while we focus our attention on the patients who need us more."

"Are you kidding? That's an insult to this woman who is about to die," said Mel.

"You believe her?"

Van Woert had that pained-worried expression on his face and nodded his head "yes." "Not only do I believe her. I actually think she will die and die soon."

"Come on, Mel! That's ridiculous!"

"Maybe not this afternoon, as she predicted, but soon. And we won't know why. And even after autopsy, we won't know why. Put her under close observation.

Tell Nurse Petersen I want vital signs every 15 minutes. I hope the disease sends clues. Until it does, we wait. And while we are waiting, she may die. But God knows why."

"Mel, she is just emotional about not getting attention. That's what Cotzias thought. And he proved it with the Darvon. The headache went away without her popping the pill."

Before Mel could answer, Nurse Petersen appeared in the doorway. From her look, we knew what had happened.

A few days later, in the watering hole where we doctors got our after-rounds coffee, a tired-looking Cotzias stretched his arm above his head, parted his lips as if to yawn, but drew them down into a smile.

"One good thing about the dead: they make room. Beatrice is dead. No question she predicted her death. I don't know how they do it, but they do. The autopsy showed nothing, right, Mel?"

Mel nodded, and that was that.

Beatrice was the first patient who did that to me, and there have been others. One man told me why he was going to die: his death was going to be the punishment for having given the boat keys to his son.

Baylor College of Medicine
The Father and the Boat Keys

Me: "I don't understand."

He: "My wife told me not to give him the keys. There was a storm coming up in the Gulf, and it would be too dangerous to go boating. The boat went down. His friend told me the last thing he saw was my son screaming for help. Watch Doc, my right hand will start to shrink, and then everything will fall apart."

Me: "Right hand?"

He: "That was the hand I used to give my son the keys. That is where the punishment will start."

Me: "Don't be ridiculous. If something goes wrong, come to me, and we will try to fix it."

He: "I'll let you see me go down. But no tests or treatments."

Within three months, that man was dead. The dwindling disease started as he said it would in his right hand and progressed rapidly. Dwindles is a very serious condition that is always fatal. What mechanism enables a person to self-destruct is not known. There must be some way the brain can make the body die. I have seen mention of dwindles in the medical literature. But now it is called the fragility syndrome. People just start getting fragile, and nothing can save them. Current thinking is it is a total body mitochondrial failure due to unknown causes.

Columbia-Presbyterian Hospital
My Mother Predicted Her Death

Much to my regret, mom predicted her death. When she was in Harkness Pavilion at Columbia-Presbyterian Medical Center, she would order gourmet dinners brought into her room, and we ate together. The food was much better than what was served at Bard Hall, the dining room for medical students, and mom and I enjoyed each other's company. One night, as I was working my way through a nice filet mignon, mom announced, "Mickey, tonight I am going to die."

"Mom, don't talk like that. It sounds ridiculous."

"No, I know I am going to die tonight, and I am trying to say goodbye."

At that point, I erupted and screamed at her. "Cut it out. You are not going to die. The doctors still have tricks up their sleeves. You are being ridiculous, and I won't stand for it."

"Mickey, I am going to die, and instead of sympathy, all I get is abuse. Don't be a pest!"

I kissed her on the forehead and left in a huff. I wish I could go back and tell her how sorry I am, tell her I just didn't want her to die, tell her that I love her. But I can't. It's too late. Dying is never easy, whatever we wish to think. Dying is especially hard for those who are doing the dying. The memory of mom's death provokes pain and tears. Why did she have to undergo five years of such colossal suffering? It wasn't fair. Come to think on it, the whole situation on this planet is wrong. It is wrong for people to die. It is wrong for people to suffer.

In the hallway, I met Doctor Cosgrove, mom's internist. He told me that mom was in bad shape, "It's the end of the trail. We're out of ideas. The disease is too strong. She will die soon. Maybe even tonight."

She died that night.

And now I have to live with the fact that the last words my mother said to me were: "Don't be a pest!" Come to think of it, it is good advice.

As I became more experienced, I learned that some patients somehow can and do predict their deaths. There are, I believe, two great systems for understanding human nature. One is psychiatry, and the other is literature. In the *Chanson de Roland*, Gawain is asked, "Ah, good my lord, think you then so soon to die?" Gawain answers, "I tell you that I shall not live two days."

Gawain was right!

Old Medical Literature is Instructive about Power to Induce Your Own Death

Much of the old medical literature is lost to modern eyes because it has not been put in the electronic databases. The solution to that problem is to visit the stacks and pull down the old journals and read. In one article, a doctor sutured a cat's anus closed. The cat got very sick, and the researcher measured progressively increasing blood ammonia levels. The cat died. Conclusion: an open anus is necessary but not sufficient for life, and blood ammonia rises if the anus is closed. The possible mechanism of death is ammonia intoxication.

In another ancient article, President Grant's physician gives it for his opinion Grant's cancer of the mouth is due to "smoking too many cigars." Indeed, many articles in the 1920-1940 journals claim smoking cigarettes causes lung cancer! Fancy that! One article in Science showed that patients whose hospital window looks out over a garden recover faster than those whose hospital window looks over a parking lot. This proves a room with a good view counts.

And then there is the pencil of happiness study. A pencil is used to induce facial expression. If the pencil is held in the teeth, the face takes on the appearance of a smile and the brain scans show that the brain gets happy, and, of course, the person gets happy as well. If the same pencil is held in the lips, the facial muscles assume positions that resemble sadness, and, lo and behold, the brain scans show the changes associated with sadness, and the person tends to feel sad as well. In other words, the brain takes clues from the position of the facial muscles, a form of bottom-up behavior modification. Therefore, smile, smile, smile, if you wish to get happy.

Patients Predict Their Own Death

The article I like best comes from *Archives of Neurology and Psychiatry* 36 (1936), wherein a Hindu doctor gets permission to conduct what would today be a forbidden experiment. The doctor convinces a prisoner to permit himself to be bled to death instead of hung. The condemned convict is strapped to a bed, blindfolded, and cut superficially in arms and legs. Meanwhile, four bags of water are set up and start to drip into pans. First, the drips come fast and loud and then gradually taper off. Finally, there is silence. The prisoner appears to have fainted, but on closer inspection is found dead despite having lost no more than four drops of blood. The article's title tells it all: "Killed by the imagination."

> **Lesson:** There is a connection, the mechanism of which is as yet undiscovered between the brain and body such that the brain may extinct the body.

Baylor College of Medicine
Patients Who Predict Their Recovery

The reverse is true. People can will themselves to live. There are patients who had serious progressive diseases that seemed hopeless (ALS for example) who have willed themselves to recover and did recover. Experience dictates the will to live is one of the most important prognostic factors in any illness. I could relate events about such people who had supposedly fatal diseases yet recovered on their own. But why bother? No one would believe me.

Whoa! Don't believe me that no one would believe me? See what you think about the following patient named Eve. See if you believe in her recovery as an example of the importance of the power of the will to live.

Eve

She had been the director of a hospital in Arizona when she developed amyotrophic lateral sclerosis. Her neurologist referred her to me in the hope something might be done, or the diagnosis might be wrong, and a more treatable condition discovered.

Her general examination and her neurological examination indicated the well-known and classical findings of amyotrophic lateral sclerosis. The laboratory examination, which included electromyograms, muscle and nerve biopsies, and spinal fluid tests, confirmed the diagnosis.

Eve had a fatal disease and was told that fact. Her blood gases, which measured the oxygen content of the blood and the carbon dioxide content of the blood, showed deficient oxygenation and excessive carbon dioxide, indicating that Eve had respiratory deficiency due to weak muscles. My advice was for her to go on a respirator to support her life. Otherwise, her future would be very short, indeed. She refused. I advised her to at least consider having respiratory assist during sleep so that she wouldn't die during sleep. She refused and was discharged from the hospital. Prognosis: grim.

Two years later, Eve called and asked to be readmitted to the hospital for examinations to prove that her disease was in remission or had disappeared. The examinations and the tests were now normal. My impression was that the disease, amyotrophic lateral sclerosis, had disappeared. But how? And why? Here is Eve's take on the situation:

"I hated my job. There was no way I could continue as a hospital director. The stress was enormous, and I was being blamed for things I had no control over. The disease represented a convenient and honorable way out of a terrible situation, and I was grateful to get the disease because it got me out of the job I hated.

"After I consulted you, I knew I was about to die, so I founded a tarantology club—"

"A what?"

"Tarantology—a name derived from tarantula and indicating, having been bitten by the spider, I was about to die."

"You made up the name?"

"I'm not sure. I think so. Everything changes once you have a fatal disease. It's like you have stepped through the looking glass, and you are now in a different world.

"I went around the country, lecturing on how I was facing my death with equanimity."

"With equanimity? Meaning what?"

"That I accepted my fate. One day in New York, at the Plaza Hotel, just before I was to go on and deliver my lecture about how well I had adjusted to the idea of dying, I caught my image in the mirror and addressed the mirror image directly pointing a finger at myself: "Eve, you hypocrite, you are a liar and a fraud. You don't want to die. You want to live."

"That day, I didn't give my talk. Instead, I spent the next two weeks in that room. I am not sure what happened there or why, but I think I was psychotic and having visual and auditory hallucinations. My food was brought to the room, but aside from that, there was no contact with the outside world. At the end of the two weeks, I emerged from the cocoon with a new view of myself and my illness. My new self knew I wanted sex, both with men and with women. The insight into the illness was I had created the illness to get me out of the job I hated. I accepted the illness as the cost of getting out of work.

"My new self-bought a van, and I got a woman lover and a man lover to travel around the country with me. We had lots of fun, and my lovers were told this was my last hurrah. I was about to die. And yes, I paid them for their services. They were nice to me and sincerely loved me, but they did get paid.

"About three months into the mission, I noticed my muscles were getting stronger, and I was able to do things that I could not do before. I had never hoped to cure myself. That was, I thought, out of the question, but that was what was happening, and that was what happened. I believe there is some kind of mechanism by which the brain can make you sick and by the same power can make you well. My case shows both."

> **Lesson:** There are more things in heaven and earth than are dreamt of. Eve seemed to have amyotrophic lateral sclerosis, but it is possible that she didn't. The tests for that disease are all indirect and reflect poor function of motor neurons. She could have had something that for all intents and purposes looked like amyotrophic lateral sclerosis but actually was something else that our current state of the art failed to recognize. That "something else" was recoverable. On the other hand, she could have, by mechanisms presently unknown, engineered her recovery by changing her lifestyle, recognizing her true self, and eliminating the need for the disease the way a neurotic patient can eliminate the need for neurotic signs and symptoms by resolving the underlying conflicts.

> **Lesson:** If the greater thing is possible, then the lesser thing is also possible.

If patients can will their death and the time thereof, and if they can will not to die and will their recovery, then it should be possible for people to delay their death. Negative life events do predispose to fatality. Meaningful events may postpone death. Patients enter some kind of idea they would like to postpone death until the arrival of a special occasion, like a birthday, a wedding, an anniversary, a religious holiday, and the like. More Jews (especially the men) die the week after Passover than the week before it. More deaths occur on Monday after the weekend of relaxation and fun than during the whole weekend itself. There are twice as many coronary deaths on Monday as there are during any other weekday. The phenomenon is true for the Harvest Moon Festival for Chinese women. For them, during this gigantically important celebration of elderly women, death is postponed for the entire week. This is followed by a surge of deaths the week after the holiday.

The Curious Case of Aunt Joan

My aunt Joan was at death's door for over a year. She required 24/7 nursing care to keep her going. Joan vowed she would not die until her nephew, namely me, came to say goodbye. Telephone conversations were not enough. I had to visit. And I did. Joan and I had an important personal relation because she was the youngest of my 10 aunts. I loved Joan, and she loved me.

Ethel and I visited, and I showed Joan my Irish passport, proving I was an Irish citizen, something Joan had helped engineer.

Two hours after we left, Joan died as she said she would. The nurses were flabbergasted. They had taken care of Joan in Joan's home for over a year and had not noted any change in Joan's physical or mental condition before, during, or after my visit. And yet, Joan had not only predicted her death but also had confirmed the prediction by actually dying.

Baylor College of Medicine
Mister Harvey

Talking about Eve reminds me of Mister Harvey, who did have amyotrophic lateral sclerosis. I never got to know Mister Harvey because, at the time I was asked to see him, he was in the last stages of the disease, unable to chew, swallow, talk, or breathe. He was in Touro Infirmary, a charitable, not-for-profit, faith-based, community hospital in the Garden District of New Orleans. Touro Clinic was founded in 1852 by Judah Touro, a Jewish Philanthropist.

Patients Predict Their Own Death

Wow! The care Mister Harvey was receiving was marvelous. He was surrounded by an army of concerned nurses, physical therapists, and local doctors. The respirator care was particularly good, and Mister Harvey's lungs were in excellent shape, although he had not been able to breathe on his own for months.

Someone, I think Mister Harvey's aunt or his bodyguard or both, told me Mister Harvey was the last descendant of the last Exchequer of King Louis XVI of France, and Mister Harvey owned lots of land in Louisiana and in France and Spain, and Mister Harvey was a billionaire. Furthermore, Harvey, a census-designated place in Jefferson Parish on the west bank of the Mississippi River close to New Orleans, was named after his ancestors—Harvey, Louisiana, elevation three feet above sea level.

I agreed with the diagnosis. But I disagreed with the appraisal that Mister Harvey was not conscious. Some of the consulting neurologists from Tulane bet the electroencephalogram would show brain death. But I knew they were wrong because Mister Harvey was able to obey my commands. When I asked him to look left, he moved his eyes that way, and when I asked him to look right, he looked right.

"If you know Morse Code, move your eyes right." He did. Eye muscles are preserved in amyotrophic lateral sclerosis to the very end, as they were preserved here in Mister Harvey. That was classical. And, of course, the electroencephalogram was normal.

So, engineers at Tulane set up devices that read eye movement in one direction as a dot and eye movement in the other direction as a dash. A kind of ticker tape converted the dots and dashes into letters, so anyone at the bedside could read what Mister Harvey had to say. The whole arrangement was brilliant, an engineering coup. This situation greatly pleased Mister Harvey, who was now able to manage his businesses and to tell the nurses when he needed to be turned or when he wanted his nose scratched and so forth. The setup greatly pleased his aunt, who now was back in communication with her nephew. This pleasant situation continued until the eye movements began to fail. Eventually, the eyes stopped moving, and again, Mister Harvey was out of communication. Again, I was consulted.

Imagine what it is like if you can't move. You have an itch, and you can't scratch it. As the itch spreads, you can't turn your head or raise eyebrows or honk or whatnot to tell someone to scratch the itch for you. If the itch is bad enough, maybe your eyes will tear, and the tear will run down your face, and you won't be able to wipe it away. Imagine you can't even swallow your own saliva, and you can't get someone to suction it away from your windpipe. You feel things alright—itches, cramps, a full bladder—but you can't do anything. You can't move. You are trapped in your body. Ugh!

Finger examination of the rectum showed that Mister Harvey could still contract and relax his rectal sphincter muscle on my command. That is a peculiar feature of this disease. The very last muscle under voluntary control was still working—his rectal sphincter muscle was still under voluntary control. So, a small balloon probe was inserted in Mister Harvey's rectum, and he was able to send dots and dashes again.

The visits to Mister Harvey took place on Fridays. The routine was after work at Baylor, I would fly to New Orleans and round on Mister Harvey. After visiting Mister Harvey, Mister Harvey's bodyguard and I would then have a delicious dinner at the Commander's Palace, a famous restaurant also in the Garden District of New Orleans. And after that, the bodyguard and I would make rounds in the French Quarter. There is always something going on there, and most of it will remain unpunished.

One Friday night, under the bodyguard's protection, I entered a bar on Bourbon Street. The bartender gave the high sign, and the bodyguard and I passed behind the bar and down a flight of stairs to a darkly lit basement. There in the dark, dank, dreary gloom, there were grown men tied to iron rings on the wall. Most of them had nothing on, except one elderly man had underpants or a diaper. In the gloom, I couldn't tell which.

Each man was attended by a beautiful woman dressed in black leather who was shouting at their man-victim and whipping him with some kind of whip. Whew! You don't forget a scene like that. It is something I would have never ventured to see if I had not been protected by an armed guard. The range of human behaviors is enormous. For some reason, those men needed and wanted to be punished and were willing to pay for the service.

Talking about pay reminds me I did get paid to see Mister Harvey. On the very first visit, without my asking or, for that matter, even thinking about pay, Mister Harvey's aunt wrote out a check for $2,000 and handed it to me asking if that was enough.

It was.

I Failed Mister Harvey

Eventually, the rectal sphincter failed, as we thought it would, and Mister Harvey was again out of communication. With the Tulane doctors and engineers, we tried to train Mister Harvey to send dots and dashes via adjusting his alpha rhythm in his brainwaves. This is possible to do voluntarily. I know that for sure, because I can do it. I can change my electroencephalogram to alpha by suspending all thoughts, and I can let it slip back again to normal by starting to think. So, at least theoretically, it would be possible to send a dot and dash by changing the alpha rhythm in the brainwaves. If we could teach Mister Harvey to do that, he would be back with us.

Jesus, I wish I had thought of that sooner, so we could have started Mister Harvey's brainwave training before he lost his rectal sphincter tone. But alas, Mister Harvey was now out of communication, unable to control his brainwaves for communication, and I was out of ideas. Imagine what it must be like to be completely helpless, unable to move a single muscle, unable to communicate with anyone! A prisoner in your own body! Not good! Why, oh why, was I not thinking ahead?

Mister Harvey developed pneumonia and was treated with small doses of penicillin.

He died. His aunt made a donation to my research and offered the use of Mister Harvey's apartment on Trocadéro in the 16th arrondissement Paris, which I never got around to using because on sabbatical in 1990, Ethel and I had our own apartment on Rue de la Croix-Nivert in the 15th arrondissement at Rue de la Convention.

Lesson: It pays to think ahead of the power curve and prepare for future developments that are likely to occur. I knew the rectal muscles would fail and should have prepared Mr. Harvey in advance with brainwave training.

The next patient illustrates an important point about supposedly fatal conditions. Sometimes, the diagnosis of a fatal disease merely reflects the ignorance of the doctors and not the disease itself. Wrong diagnosis may lead to wrong management and a wrong result.

Tableau Twenty-Five:

Coma Due to Kidney Failure?

New York Hospital, Cornell Medical Center
Coma Due to Kidney Failure

One of the first things that you do when you rotate on a medical service as an intern is to get acquainted with the patients who will be your responsibility.

On ward G3H3 at the New York Hospital, I was told by the resident there was a patient in a coma that had been assigned to me. She was a 54-year-old woman admitted to the hospital for evaluation of polycystic kidney disease. This is a disease in which there are multiple cysts in the kidney, and the cysts may cause problems with kidney function.

"She won't be much trouble because, within a few days of her admission, she became very sleepy and weak. After a week in the hospital, she became somnolent, and after two weeks in the hospital, she lapsed into coma. Don't bother with her. She will be dead soon."

My first question was, "What was the cause of the coma?"

With straight faces, the two residents (the junior resident and the senior resident) told me, "Renal failure."

My next question, "What's the BUN?"

BUN is an abbreviation for blood urea nitrogen. It is a nice measure of kidney function. Usually, the BUN is 20 or below. If it rises above 20, it means the patient has lost over 80% of their kidney function. The degree of elevation of the BUN is roughly proportional to the amount of kidney failure. Asking about the BUN was a reasonable question, considering the patient was in a coma supposedly caused by renal failure. Her BUN was 86.

I exclaimed, "Holy Cow! A BUN of 86, and the patient is in a coma?"

Merle Sande, the senior medical resident who many years later became a very famous physician in San Francisco (but who is now dead), said, "We see it."

Yep. They see it. That "we see it" sent up a red flag. Whenever you hear "We see it" it usually means they don't see it, and they never have seen it. It usually means they are covering ignorance—vast ignorance.

Ignorance is not altogether bad, especially if the ignorance involves knowing that you don't know something.

That was great. I love a case like this, where the powers that be have already written off the patient. There isn't anything to lose. And there is the possibility of a big win. I decided to put on my mantle as the patron saint of the lost.

Third question, but this question was to myself: "Why was she in a coma?"

The Quest for an Answer

Because I didn't know anything about coma, I got books about it, and I read, and read, and read. *Coma and Stupor* by Plum and Posner was the best book on the subject and was clinically oriented and based on practical experience at the bedside. Working my way through it, I discovered that there were a number of things on physical examination that gave hints about the cause of coma. What the book said to do—I did.

The patient had no reflexes, so I couldn't lateralize a specific cerebral lesion. She did have pupils that were round, regular, and equal that responded to light. According to the book, if a patient has round, regular, and equal pupils that respond to light, the cause of the coma is metabolic. That is, if the pupils look like that—round and regular and respond to light, the coma is not due to a structural lesion in the brain. It is due to a metabolic defect, something chemical that is preventing brain cells from functioning properly. This is important because if the metabolic cause of coma could be discovered, it might be reversible. Bingo! This patient might have a reversible coma!

In a general sense, renal failure would be considered a metabolic cause of coma. The trouble was that the BUN was too low for renal failure to do that. My patient had renal insufficiency, not renal failure. Therefore, renal failure as the cause of coma in my patient was ruled out—excluded. It was not possible. She didn't have it. That left a great big question mark. What was causing the metabolic coma? The previous diagnosis was wrong. I knew that, but I still didn't know what was causing the coma. No one knew. Some thought they knew. But they were wrong. I, at least knew, I didn't know, and I knew they were wrong about the cause of coma. That put me ahead of the crowd. The next question was: what to do?

What Do You Do When You Don't Know What to Do?

I copied into the order book requests for blood tests for every known metabolic cause of coma. I just copied it straight from the Plum and Posner coma book into the order book, drew the blood, and sent off all the blood samples to the laboratory. There were 27 blood tests looking for possible metabolic causes of coma. They ranged from drug overdoses to severe hypothyroidism, adrenal insufficiency, ammonia intoxication, electrolyte imbalance, and so forth. Whew! I was trying to cover all the bets.

All the tests came back normal except for the serum magnesium, which returned elevated at 15 mEq/L. What did that mean? No one seemed to know. Not my attending. Not my residents. Not my fellow interns—I mean—my fellow assistant physicians. There were no interns at the New York Hospital. We were assistant physicians. We were all physicians, however, freshly minted. So, when the patients asked, "Are you an intern?" we truthfully replied, "No, sir, I am an assistant physician."

Back to the Coma Book

No help there. That great book failed to explain what the elevated magnesium meant and what to do about it. So, back to the medical library for a few hours. Thank God I stumbled across two review articles about magnesium. Physicians who write review articles are the unsung heroes of our time. There is little honor or academic credit for writing a review because it isn't original research, but review articles are precious gems of information for newly minted doctors who want to know what's what. Unlike the stuff you get on the internet, library information has been vetted by a responsible intelligence operating in a professional culture and, for the most part, operating outside a commercial culture.

"The only thing you absolutely have to know is the location of the library."

Albert Einstein

One review article was about hypermagnesemia—that is excessive blood levels of magnesium—and the other article was about hypomagnesemia—that is levels of magnesium in the blood that are too low.

Bingo! The review article said that magnesium blood levels of 15 mEq/L cause coma. The article went on to say that the most common cause of increased magnesium in the blood was excessive administration of magnesium to a patient who had renal insufficiency. Bingo again! This patient did have renal insufficiency. Now I just had to find out where she was getting the magnesium from.

Mystery Solved

When the patient had been admitted to the ward, she complained of epigastric distress, which the doctors thought was due to acid indigestion. She was given Maalox every four hours to neutralize stomach acid. When she started getting weak and tired and couldn't swallow anymore, they put down a tube from her nose into her stomach. And get this, the nurses had been flushing Maalox down the (nasogastric) tube every four hours ever since. Maalox has magnesium hydroxide and is a common source of magnesium toxicity according to the review article.

Great! That's the probable diagnosis. Coma due to magnesium intoxication. Now the question was what to do. Multiple treatments were available. The basic idea was to lower the blood level of magnesium, to decrease the effect of magnesium on the nervous system, or both.

I called the renal service in consultation. Perhaps they could use dialysis to get the magnesium levels down. Perhaps they would have some other idea on how to handle the problem. No dice. They were very busy with very sick patients, and they also didn't understand coma of this magnitude and thought that it could not possibly be related to the renal insufficiency, as the BUN was only 86. They knew a BUN of 86 indicated sufficient renal function to support life and reasonable health and consciousness. Therefore, dialysis, they felt, was not indicated for this degree of renal insufficiency. How's that for restricted thinking! I wanted them to remove magnesium by dialysis, not bother with the BUN. But they had never heard of such a thing.

Jesus Christ. They missed the point.

No dice. Dialysis is out.

More Work in the Library

There were other treatments. Administration of calcium intravenously was said to reverse the adverse effect of magnesium immediately. However, giving calcium intravenously had the possible side effect of arresting the heart. I didn't want to take that risk. Discretion is the better part of valor. So, I simply told the nurses to stop the Maalox. That was my major treatment for this patient. I wrote in the order book the Maalox was to be stopped. The next part of the treatment was to keep my hands in my pocket, watch and wait, and repeatedly check the blood magnesium to make sure it was coming down.

Soon, the serum magnesium levels declined to 10 mEq/L. The patient regained consciousness! She woke up in a daze, amnesic for all of her hospital stay. At 9 mEq/L she walked! She was weak and unsteady when she walked, but she did walk and was even able to go to the bathroom by herself, a return of function noted and praised by the nursing staff.

Coma Due to Kidney Failure?

At 7 mEq/L, her deep tendon reflexes returned, and at 4 mEq/L she and everybody else who had seen her on admission to the hospital said that she was back to her usual state of health. Throughout this period, the BUN remained stable at 80 to 86.

Here's What I Learned

Alterations of magnesium concentrations profoundly affect nerve and muscle function. The biological role of magnesium is well-known, and magnesium is, in fact, the body's fourth most abundant cation and the second most abundant intracellular ion, second only to potassium. When you get some ion like this in that kind of concentration, it has to be important, and it has to be contributing to making life. Any alteration of magnesium (too high or too low) or potassium causes trouble. Somewhere down the line, I will tell you a real sad story about too much potassium in the blood but not now.

Magnesium maintains activation of literally hundreds of enzymatic reactions in the body, including those involved in phosphate transfer, glycolysis, and ion transport. Half of the body's magnesium resides in bone, but high concentrations exist in the liver, brain, and muscle. The usual serum concentration ranges between 1.6 and 2.1 mEq/L, one-third of which is bound to serum proteins. Serum magnesium levels like those of potassium do not always reflect the actual content in tissues, and the concentration of magnesium in cerebral spinal fluid exceeds the serum concentration by 1.8 mEq/L, meaning more than twice the diffusible fraction of serum magnesium must be actively transported into the cerebral compartment across the blood-brain barrier.

People eat about 40 mEq magnesium daily, mainly in meats and vegetables. Intestinal absorption occurs, rapidly followed by urinary excretion of excess amounts. If the kidney is damaged, the magnesium taken in cannot be excreted and begins to pile up in the blood.

In modern medicine, magnesium salts are used as cathartics or central nervous system depressants, as in the treatment of toxemia of pregnancy or in control of eclamptic convulsions. High doses of magnesium block neuromuscular transmission, interfering with the calcium-dependent release of acetylcholine and decreasing the sensitivity to acetylcholine in the muscle membrane. That explains why the patient was weak and why she didn't have reflexes during the time her magnesium blood levels were elevated. The paralytic effect can be reversed by administering calcium, by reducing the magnesium levels, or by increasing the effectiveness of small amounts of acetylcholine, released by preventing the acetylcholine esterase with any anticholinesterase drug, such as the agents used in the treatment of myasthenia gravis.

Clinical features for hypermagnesemia depend on serum level of ionized magnesium. Lower than normal plasma protein concentrations and acidosis increase ionized magnesium, and therefore the clinical symptoms will be augmented. This is especially significant in renal insufficiency.

Usually, two events are required before excessive magnesium accumulates in the blood. First, you must have an increased intake of magnesium, as was the case with this woman who received magnesium, by mouth at first when she could swallow, and then when she could not swallow, magnesium was given by nasogastric tube. Second, you must have decreased excretion of magnesium because of (you guessed it) kidney trouble.

Thus, this patient was a classic example of the result of partial renal failure and magnesium overload. Aside from the renal failure, fatal magnesium intoxication has followed magnesium sulfate enemas and as a complication of magnesium therapy of eclampsia. In eclampsia, both mother and child are at risk because magnesium crosses the placenta barrier. Children born to mothers treated with intravenous magnesium salts may develop severe paralysis due to excessive magnesium in their blood. The situation is not helped by the fact the kidney of the newborn human is not able to excrete magnesium efficiently. Naturally, the doctors can reverse the neuromuscular effects of excess magnesium by appropriate therapy. Since the premature infant kidney often excretes magnesium slowly, clinically significant prolonged hypermagnesemia does occur in this setting, and this should be looked for in a floppy infant born to a mother who was treated for eclampsia with magnesium salts. Such children manifest varying degrees of weakness, ranging from mild loss of muscle tone to quadriplegia (that is paralysis of arms and legs) with respiratory failure and multiple cardiac arrhythmias.

Therapy of Hypermagnesemia

Mild cases respond to simply stopping the magnesium salts the patient was receiving and watching the serum level decline. In severe cases, especially those with cardiac toxicity, intravenous calcium salts reduce the myocardial toxicity immediately. The calcium salt should be given slowly, intravenously under electrocardiograph control to avoid the arrest of the heart. Glucose and insulin can also be used in the same way you would use glucose and insulin to flush magnesium into the cell, but you could also use the same treatment to flush potassium into cells, temporarily reducing the serum levels of both potassium and magnesium. The treatment of choice for sick infants with hypermagnesemia is exchange transfusion.

Coma Due to Kidney Failure?

General Comments

This interesting and important patient taught me some lessons and not just about magnesium:

> **Lesson:** There is a big difference between knowing what is wrong with the patient and thinking you know what is wrong with the patient.

The resident and the other people on the service were sincere in believing the patient was in coma from renal failure. It was only on further investigation, attempting to get to the real cause of the problem, the real cause of the coma was discovered. Along the way, I learned a great deal about the role of magnesium in human physiology, and I immodestly state, at that moment in time, I knew more about magnesium than any other person at the New York Hospital, Cornell Medical center. In fact, I probably knew more about magnesium than anyone in New York City, and perhaps even in New York State. Such knowledge will save the life of another woman patient, as you will read about soon.

> **Lesson:** Luck plays a role in survival.

The patient was lucky. I took an interest in her problem. I was lucky to stumble across the review articles on magnesium pretty much by accident. The old days did not have electronic indexes or the internet. Trips to the library searching for specific information were largely hit or miss. I like to think it was Irish luck that saved her. God gives the Irish tremendous luck to make up for their tremendous stupidity and to level the playing field against the Jews. On the other hand, there was more to this than luck because, after all, I was in the library trying to solve the patient's problem. It was not luck that a medical intern, in those days, at the New York Hospital, Cornell Medical Center had the time to do library research work on his patient's problem. In those days, I had the time because I needed only three hours sleep. My intern partner and I learned we could survive on only three hours sleep if we managed to get a half hour nap in the afternoon.

Lesson: When we hear someone say, "I see it," we had better not believe them unless their statement is backed up by evidence that is relevant and adequate. Adequate evidence should be sufficient in number, kind, and weight to justify the conclusion. Otherwise, we had better conclude they "don't see it," and what they think they know is mere conjecture. We, they, or someone, before the patient croaks, had better start looking for the real answer.

Final Diagnosis

The correct diagnosis led to the correct treatment, which saved the patient's life. The mission of medicine was fulfilled, as the survival of the individual patient is one of the many missions of medicine.

The Point is Doctors Need Time and Energy to Work Out Solutions for Hard Cases

Attention reader: don't doze off. I am not telling you about this patient to crow about how I saved her life. That's not the point. Here's the point: I ask you this. Is it likely under the present conditions of rushed medical care, this woman would have survived her magnesium-induced intoxication? Is it likely a harassed modern doctor would have had the energy, time, or enthusiasm to work on this patient's problem the way I did? Regrettably, I think there are lots of people out there who need special medical help and are not getting it. In this day and age, if your problem is not simple and straightforward and easily solvable by application of a cookbook algorithm, you might be in trouble, sometimes big trouble. Under the present system of medical payment, thinking about and studying the patient's problem is not well compensated, but doing a procedure on the patient is well compensated. Therefore, there is a tendency to do less thinking and more procedures and more tests.

Missed Diagnosis

Dante said that in order to appreciate the good, we should mention some things that are not so good. Not so good was my mistake in taking care of a patient with fever and skin rash.

She was in her early 40s, a mother of two girls, and lived in Kew Gardens, Queens. She seemed to have some kind of autoimmune disease, according to the rheumatology specialists, and she didn't have an infectious disease according to the infectious disease consultants. Her private doctor, who was both a doctor and a minister, visited every day and felt strongly this was a serious infection that needed treatment with tetracycline. Since I, as intern on the case, controlled the order book, it fell on me to decide what treatment was needed. Following the recommendation of rheumatologists, I started the patient on prednisone. Within a day, she was worse and had to be admitted to the intensive care unit, where I tried to take care of her deteriorating condition. The rate of worsening alarmed her, her family, and me. Her kidneys were failing, and so were her lungs; blood pressure was dropping, and she needed more and more support (intravenous fluids, nasal oxygen, norepinephrine, and so forth) to keep her going. She cried when I tried to explain we were doing everything we could think of to get her condition under control. I felt like crying too but managed to hold back. A cold sweat ran down my back as I left the ICU. It looked like my patient was pre-cool. ("Going to cool" was the New York Hospital slang expression for going to die. "Pre-cool" meant about to die. "He cooled last night" meant the patient died last night.)

Rheumatology advised increasing the prednisone, and her private physician insisted the prednisone be stopped and tetracycline started. The infectious disease people laughed at the private doc's idea. They pooh-poohed the tetracycline saying, "If he thought it was an infection, why not use a much more powerful antibiotic like vancomycin or high-dose penicillin?"

Clearly, they, the members of the full-time faculty, thought the minister/doctor was a "turkey" (lousy doctor), who probably should never have gotten privileges at the New York Hospital. "They should take his license away. Or he should stick to religion since he doesn't know medicine."

What to do? That's the question. Believe whom and what?

Sunday Night the Trouble Started

The private doctor/minister snuck into the intensive care unit and wrote an order for tetracycline, an order, which, on advice of the rheumatologists and infectious disease experts, I canceled on Monday morning.

Minister/doctor: "Patten, you have to believe me. Her life is in your hands. Can't you see the present approach did not work, is not working, and will not work in the future? God wants you to countersign my order for tetracycline."

Rheumatology service: "Bernie, you have to believe us. Her life is in your hands. She has severe autoimmune disease. If you stop the treatments, she will die. She is already at death's door."

Infectious disease service: "No way this is an infection, and no way tetracycline will do any good. In fact, the opposite is true. It may make her situation worse. Her kidneys are almost shot, so tetra will bump them off."

And so, a war started with the private doctor/minister coming in the middle of the night and writing an order for tetracycline, and the infectious disease people telling me to cancel the order, which I always did. Rheumatology seemed to know what they were doing, and they were sure the patient had an autoimmune disease. So, I continued their treatment recommendations.

One Monday afternoon, the minister came to talk. He was dressed like a priest—all in black with a white collar. And he talked in that stilted, suave way that ministers talk. He explained he thought this was some kind of infection.

"How do you know for sure?"

"I have faith in God. The idea of infection and that tetracycline was the correct treatment just popped into my mind. It could have been a message from God, but I'm not sure. It could have come from some deep unconscious reasoning I can't explain. Other than that, I admit there is no scientific evidence to support my conviction that tetracycline is needed. Please, Doctor Patten, save her life. Give her tetracycline, 500mg four times a day for the next two weeks. A trial of that antibiotic will do no harm."

"That's not what I was told."

Rheumatologists said, "Tetracycline might worsen the already failing kidneys and will worsen her failing liver." The infectious disease team said, "Ditto."

Six blood cultures were negative—that is the blood grew no organisms. So, I held off on antibiotics and stuck with immune suppression for what I thought was a rapidly progressing autoimmune disease.

The trouble was no one had ever seen or heard of an autoimmune disease that progresses so fast, and no one, not even the rheumatologists, could actually pin a name on what they thought was my patient's disease. In other words, there wasn't a specific diagnosis, just a theory of what was wrong. That ignorance was the red flag that should have made me realize that the case had to be rethought. We were on the wrong track, but I didn't know it. I was too stupid to recognize the truth.

Coma Due to Kidney Failure?

Result

She died.

A Tragedy of Shakespearean Proportions

Ugh!

The autopsy showed the woman died of rickettsialpox: Kew Garden fever.

Lesson: Always get the autopsy.

Lesson: When things go wrong, examine the circumstances, and try to find out why.

The only medicine that would have saved her was tetracycline! Rickettsial diseases can look like autoimmune diseases, but treatment with prednisone would just worsen the infection by lowering the patient's immunity. That's what happened. Tetracycline would have killed the bacterium causing the disease and given the patient an excellent chance to recover. The organism is a sort of half-breed that has features of bacteria and features of a virus. The rickettsial organism usually remains inside of cells and thus is very hard to detect with routine blood cultures and the usual antibiotics. In this disease, tetracycline would have been the drug of choice.

Stupid me! I completely missed the diagnosis. I believed the half-truths and bull-shit of the rheumatologists and infectious disease experts. I even had read Berton Rouechè's short story about the original outbreak of Kew Garden fever in 1946. Thus, I missed the cue in Kew. And I knew Kew Garden fever was spread by a mite that had gotten the disease from mice that hang out in the apartments of Kew Gardens, Queens. The infectious disease people had given bad advice, although they meant well, and the rheumatology people had given bad advice, although they meant well. The fact I should have paid more attention to was the dramatic worsening of the patient's clinical condition when the prednisone was started. That was the tip-off that I was on the wrong path and should have backtracked.

What did I learn from this catastrophe?

> **Lesson:** Remember, you are never as smart as you think you are.

> **Lesson:** Experts can be wrong, even when giving advice in their field.

> **Lesson:** When the patient gets worse on a treatment, it is time to rethink the entire case.

> **Lesson:** Absence of evidence is not evidence of absence. The negative blood cultures did not rule out an infection. If you see it, you believe it. If you don't see it, you don't know.

New York Hospital
A Mistake is Made; Consequently, a Patient is Dispatched to the Hereafter

My intern partner and I shared call every other night and every other weekend. On Saturdays, we made rounds together, made sure all the patients were stable, and then who was off that weekend took off and the other held the fort until Monday morning. The arrangement gave one of us a complete Sunday off every other week.

One Sunday, I got a call from my intern partner. He had slept all Saturday afternoon and all Saturday night, and on Sunday he had headed to Sunken Meadow Park on the North Shore of Long Island for a relaxing day at the beach.

Firmly fitted in a rubber tire tube, he floated out into the cold deep greenish waters of the Long Island Sound and stared up at the beautiful (light blue) robin's egg sky. At last, he could forget the job and relax.

Suddenly, he realized he had made a mistake, a terrible mistake. He had written an order for a potassium saving drug (Aldactone) for a patient who was already taking potassium chloride by mouth. That combination would lead to a sharp rise in serum potassium and arrest the heart.

He jumped off the tire tube, swam fast back to shore, ran to a phone and paged me at the New York Hospital.

He: "Bernie, get to Mrs. Dogweed on 9. Stop the potassium and check the EKG (electrocardiogram). Her serum K+ (potassium) is probably out of sight."

I sprinted up the stairs to Mrs. Dogweed's room. She was a nice grandmother-type woman, 67 years old and a little startled by my apparent alarm and my panting shortness of breath.

Me: "Nothing to worry about, Mrs. Dogweed. But I need to check your blood potassium. Nurse, send this to the lab stat (stat = statim, Latin for "right away") and have them phone the result ASAP."

Ugh! The EKG showed sharply peaked T waves—the classic sign of too much potassium. I put in an iv (intravenous line) and ran in glucose and insulin, the standard treatment. Mrs. Dogweed was still calm as a clam, but I wasn't. I was scared stiff. Dogweed was close to becoming dog shit. She was close to cardiac arrest. Jesus H. Christ, what else should be done? I didn't know.

Me to the nurses now assembled and ready to help: "Call Tom Jones (the chief medical resident) and get him here stat. Call the arrest team. We may need them."

It seemed a century, but Tom arrived within minutes. He looked at the EKG and shook his head. Nurse Petersen rushed in with the bad news: "Potassium 9.6! Extremely high! The lab says they checked it twice. They never have seen potassium that high."

And then, as if on cue, Mrs. Dogweed's eyes rolled up, and the EKG became a flat line. Tom and I went to work with CPR. The arrest team arrived and joined in.

Four hours later, and multiple zaps with the defibrillator, we were still at it when Tom called it.

Tom: "Hopeless. She's gone. Stop."

Mrs. Dogweed was dead. Dead from a little stupid thing: blood potassium too high caused by a medicine wrong for her.

Unreal. It seemed unreal. She was alive and talking just a few hours ago, and now she was dead and silent. Dead for all time. Silent for all time.

An execution had taken place. Granted, it was an honest mistake, but a patient had been prematurely dispatched to the hereafter by well-trained, good human beings who meant well. I was exhausted and heartbroken. You can imagine how terrible my intern partner felt. The fault was not his alone. The system played a role. He had been zombified from lack of sleep during 36 hours of duty and was not thinking properly.

Every drug is a potential poison in disguise. The medieval alchemist and philosopher, Paracelsus, said, "All substances are poisonous: there is none that is not a poison. The right dose distinguishes a poison and a remedy."

There is more to it than that. It has to be the right medicine, for the right reason, by the right route, at the right time, for the right patient. Friar Lawrence, in Romeo and Juliet, expressed the dual nature of medicine more poetically: "Within the infant rind of this small flower poison hath residence, and medicine power."

Water Can Be a Poison

Even water can be a poison. At Ben Taub General Hospital we had four women patients who had watched the same TV program about the need to drink eight glasses of water. For some reason, according to the daughter of one of these ladies, they thought the program said eight glasses of water eight times a day. They all developed water intoxication with low serum sodium. The low serum sodium caused a disease of the brainstem called central pontine myelinolysis, which, in turn, causes coma and arrest of brainstem function, including loss of breathing, loss of blood pressure control, and loss of heart action. The Magnetic Resonance Image showed the diagnosis exactly with loss of myelin in the central pons of the brainstem, but unfortunately, there was no effective treatment. They all died. They all died from drinking too much water!

> **Lesson:** Those potassium-sparing diuretics are good medicines that are very helpful when used properly. When not used properly, even good medicines can be poisons.

> **Lesson:** Drinking too much water can be fatal.

Coma Due to Kidney Failure?

> **Lesson:** Don't believe everything you see or hear on TV.

Talking about Mrs. Dogweed, who had a high potassium problem, reminds me of another patient who also had a high level of another metal in the blood. His name was Richard. I'll tell you about him shortly. His is a great story. But first I want to mention two other patients saved during internship.

New York Hospital, Cornell Medical Center
Cardiac Arrest

In those days, ICU was a new idea and a new invention. The idea was to have a place where those patients who needed intensive care could get it. As the assistant physician (There are no interns, remember, at the New York Hospital. We were interns alright, but our official title was assistant physician, and we were not allowed to call ourselves interns) on duty, I had to sleep in a small room next to the ICU. If an emergency arose, the nurse would wake me, and I would take care of it. These days, physicians on duty sleep in scrubs. Those days, I slept in my underpants. There was no air conditioning, so sleeping in just underpants was the rule. One night, the nurse screamed "Arrest stat!" I rushed in. A middle-aged, white-haired grandmother-type patient had arrested. Her electrocardiogram on the scope showed a flat line. The chance of getting her back was slim, very slim.

"Paddles on! Clear!"

Zaapp!

The patient's body arched up with the shock and then settled back in bed. There was a smell of ozone and the smell of burned skin. The scope showed a flat line. The normal action of the heart is initiated by an electric charge made by the sinus pacemaker. That was not in evidence, so I knew it was not working. If the sinus pacemaker fails, usually another pacer takes over. It is lower down and slower. Since there was nothing from the lower regions of the heart, I knew the nodal pacemaker was not working. When the electrical system of the heart fails, the heart can't contract, and the circulation fails, and the patient dies. Think about that! A small amount of electric current in the heart makes the difference between life and death.

"Turn up the juice to max!"

"Paddles on! Clear!"

Zaapp!

Doctors and nurses enjoy dramatic cases like this and the carnival-like atmosphere. It's even more fun when the patient comes back. Most of them don't come back. On ICU duty, I dealt with death daily, mostly in the form of attempted resuscitations that failed. Real medical scenes are quite different from what is shown on TV.

Zaapp!

Again, the upward thrust of the body with the back tightly arched. But this time, her heart came back, and she came back with it. She smiled, and then had that surprised face. Me too. I was surprised because usually the flatliners don't come back, and, in fact, most physicians would not have bothered with the paddles in this situation because a flat line is not considered a shockable rhythm. Last time I read the textbooks on this subject, I learned only ventricular tachycardia and ventricular fibrillation are shockable. But Mrs. White doesn't seem to have read the books because the shock recalled her to life. So, why did I not follow the textbook and the received standard wisdom in the case? From a practical and logical point of view, the textbooks can be wrong. It's like Pascal's wager. The upside is the patient may come back. The downside is zip: no harm could be done to a patient already sentenced to dusty death. Saint Paul, in First Corinthians, says, "The last enemy that shall be destroyed is death. For he hath put all things under his feet." In my own little way, I was fighting against death. Most doctors do. The win is temporary because all humans die eventually, but it is the best we can do under the present state of the art.

"Doctor Patten, you're in your underwear."

"Yes, Mrs. White. We had an emergency and I didn't have time to dress."

Her speech arrested. Her eyes rolled up. Her head and she flopped back in bed. The scope again showed a flat line. Zapped again at full strength, she came back and said the same exact thing:

"Doctor Patten, you're in your underwear."

"Yes, Mrs. White. We had an emergency here, and I didn't have time to dress. I regret to inform you the emergency was you. Your heart stopped, and I had to restart it. Then it stopped again, and I had to restart it. This means I must pass a wire into your heart to pace the heart. Tomorrow, they will put in a regular pacemaker. OK?"

Mrs. White seemed to nod approval and arrested again.

Coma Due to Kidney Failure?

I passed a wire into her heart via an arm vein and substituted an electrical current from a box for the sinus pacemaker that was not working. When I turned off the current, Mrs. White's heart stopped, and she lost consciousness. When I turned on the current, her heart started again, and she returned to consciousness. That proved that she needed the wire and artificial pacing. A lot of folks do.

The Worst Admission in the History of the New York Hospital

One night just before midnight, Tom Jones, the chief medical resident, called.

"Sorry to do this to you, Bernie, but you are about to get the worst admission in the history of the New York Hospital. She has terrible lupus and needs to come in. She has had over 100 admissions and is a very sick cookie. I'll send up the most recent chart with her. If you're lucky, she'll die in the elevator."

"No, Tom. Send all the charts. I always read them—all of them."

Yes, in those days, I considered it my sacred duty to read the entire medical record of the patients admitted to my care. This was part of my medical education and an important way to understand the patient's medical situation. Of course, I first took care of the immediate problems, especially the life-threatening problems, and then settled back to read the charts. In this case, the immediate problem was pneumonia and probable sepsis (infection in the blood), so I started her on blast-a-bug. Blast-a-bug was designed to kill all of the usual infective agents. Blast-a-bug consisted of high-dose penicillin (20 million units intravenously daily), methicillin (for the penicillin-resistant bugs), colistin (for the gram-negative bacteria), and amphotericin for a fungal infection. This was not overkill. This particular patient was in danger of dying of infection because she had been taking massive doses of prednisone for her systemic lupus. Prednisone is well known to suppress the immune system, which is why it was given her, but it does predispose to infection. A patient taking prednisone and seriously infected is bad news.

On examination, the patient was a 58-year-old white woman in respiratory distress. She was a physical wreck confined to bed and with all the usual signs of severe lupus erythematosus: massive skin rashes, fever, joint swelling, enlarged liver and spleen, hair loss, mucosal ulcerations, painful nodules on her legs (erythema nodosum), cold blue fingers, and cold blue toes, and so forth. She was a classic demonstration of the havoc lupus can cause. In addition, she had the serious side effects caused by prednisone treatment: moon face, central body fat, high blood pressure, and so forth. Ugh! What a mess.

But an interesting case and an interesting patient. This very nice lady was normal mentally, something almost unheard of for someone that sick with systemic lupus. That was weird. Someone this sick with lupus should be out of it. She wasn't out of it. She was mentally sharp, very sharp.

After I wrote orders and the nurses went to work, I read chart number one, thick as a novel, and in a flash, I doubled-up and fell off my chair. "Holy shit! This can't be true! But why would the chart lie?"

History (Again) Makes the Diagnosis

Five years before, she had been admitted to the hospital for treatment of a ventricular rhythm abnormality. The excessive number and kinds of extraventricular heartbeats were toned down and eventually eliminated by a medicine called Pronestyl. Pronestyl is procainamide used in those days for cardiac arrhythmias. Procainamide is a known cause of drug-induced lupus, so it was interesting to note that the patient's second admission to the hospital occurred eight weeks after the start of the procainamide. The diagnosis on the second admission was, you guessed it, lupus erythematosus.

I rushed to the bedside, turned on the light, and woke her. She shielded her eyes because the light bothered them.

"What's the matter, Doctor?"

"Have you been taking the procainamide?"

"What's that?"

"Have you been taking Pronestyl?"

"Everyday. It's for my heart."

That was another pivotal moment in my life, an epiphany. Tears came to my eyes. I couldn't help it. Even now, when I think of that scene, I cry happy tears.

Drug-induced lupus looks pretty much the same as real, naturally occurring lupus. But in drug-induced lupus, the patient is usually a white woman who gets sick in her 50s after receiving a drug that causes lupus. Most naturally occurring cases of lupus start in the early 20s to 30s. For some unknown reason, drug-induced lupus rarely involves the central nervous system or kidneys. Kidneys and central nervous system were spared in this patient, a great sign that we are dealing with the drug-induced form of lupus and not the natural wild-type disease.

There are many other drugs that cause lupus, and you can look them up on Doctor Google. The key question is what will happen if the procainamide is stopped. If it is the cause of the patient's lupus, the prognosis will be good. Within days after the withdrawal of the culprit drug, the lupus will improve, and within a few months, the disease will disappear. So, what, dear reader, will be the cornerstone of my treatment for this very sick patient?

Management

What to do?

Answer: no workup for lupus. She has had plenty of blood tests for lupus, and all are positive. No sense repeating the tests. No workup for kidney problems either. Her kidneys have always proved normal. The treatment will be (what else?): stop the procainamide, keep hands in pockets, watch, wait, and hope for improvement.

Result

Bingo! The lupus disappeared.

Sometimes medicines are just wonderful, nothing like it, and sometimes medicines are terrible, causing weird problems and side effects like systemic lupus.

The Correct Diagnosis Takes the Cake

Her family owned a bakery. Every week for the rest of my internship, they delivered a cake to whatever service I was working on. The nurses liked the cakes, and so did the other physicians. Cake is too sweet for me, so I didn't eat much.

The next patient was just as interesting in his own way.

Tableau Twenty-Six:

Another Case of Cerebral Palsy?

Baylor College of Medicine
Richard

His mother wheeled him into clinic. She is an administrator of a hospital in a suburb of Dallas. She heard about a woman who recovered from a four-year paralysis of her legs and hoped I could help her son, Richard.

And yes, the recovered patient she was talking about is the woman with a conversion reaction you already read about who had been assaulted by her pastor and cured by the talk therapy.

Richard was the result of a normal pregnancy and delivery, but he never hit mental and physical milestones on time, so he was considered, by the definition of the era, mentally retarded.

Despite handicaps, he worked full time as a stocking clerk in a supermarket until a year prior to the clinic visit when, at age 17, his thinking got worse, and he became unable to walk or work. His mother consulted three neurologists, who each told her Richard had cerebral palsy, and there was nothing to do. "There is no treatment for cerebral palsy."

On examination, Richard was a mess, with signs and symptoms of nervous system disease at every level of the neuraxis. He was demented. He drooled. He could speak only grunts and moans. His legs and arms were weak, spastic, ataxic, and he had the shakes, etc.

Mom: "I thought cerebral palsy was static. Not progressive. Richard started getting much worse at age 10 and continued to worsen until last year when he fell apart."

Me: "That's correct."

Mom: "What's correct?"

Me: "Cerebral palsy does not worsen. It is static and never progresses."

Mom: "So how do you explain Richard getting worse?"

Me: "Either he had cerebral palsy, and something else came along to make him sicker, or he never had cerebral palsy, and he had and now has that same something else making him sick and sicker."

Mom: "The other thing that bothers me is his blue eyes turned brown."

Me: "Blue eyes turned brown?"

Mom: "He used to have such beautiful blue eyes, and now they are brown."

Me: "Wow! Holy cow! That's great! I missed the eye thing. Better have another look."

I got out the ophthalmoscope and took a good look at Richard's eyes.

Me: "Bingo! We have a diagnosis. I missed something really important."

See the photo. See what I saw looking at this patient's eyes.

Richard's eyes are blue, but at the edge (the limbus) of the cornea there is a yellow-brown, copper-colored granular deposit on Descemet's membrane makes his eyes appear brown. This is none other than the famous Kayser-Fleischer ring, the best-known sign of Wilson's disease, a condition caused by a defect in copper metabolism. The ring was visible with my naked eye but looked even more impressive with my ophthalmoscope set to a +40 lens. This copper containing ring is present in every patient with neurological problems due to Wilson's disease and most patients with Wilson's disease. The ring is usually most dense, and first visible, at the upper and lower poles of the eye. When fully developed, such rings go all around, just as they did in Richard. The rings will begin to disappear after kidney transplant and after the induction of negative copper balance by penicillamine. Usually, fading will simply reduce in the reverse of the pattern of development, so the lateral margins of the cornea will lose their copper first, followed by the superior and inferior poles. I have seen the rings completely disappear in other patients undergoing therapy.

I told mom: "This is great! We are going to make Richard's brown eyes blue, and in the process, his situation will be greatly improved."

I was crying again. I wish I could stop crying over cases like this. It looks unprofessional, but I can't help it. I was all choked up and had trouble telling mom what follows.

Me: "Richard suffers from a rare disease of copper metabolism. The defect is present in every cell of his body, and it causes copper to build up in excessive amounts. Neurological symptoms are unusual before age 12, probably because insufficient copper has accumulated in the brain but can occur. I know Richard has a copper problem because I can see the copper buildup in the cornea of his eyes. That's why his blue eyes seemed to have turned brown. His eyes are still blue, but the blue color is hiding behind the brown copper."

Now mom is smiling, and then she cries too.

Richard was admitted to the Methodist Hospital for diagnosis and treatment. The characteristic laboratory feature of the disease is a low or absent serum ceruloplasmin, the blood protein that carries copper in normal people. I expected Richard's ceruloplasmin level to be zero. Normal adults have a value between 200 and 400 milligrams per liter. The absent protein is not the cause of copper accumulation. It is just a marker of the defect. Richard's ceruloplasmin was reported by the laboratory at 325, a normal value.

Oh No! The Lab Test Fails to Confirm the Clinical Diagnosis

Ugh! What do we do now?

The most important laboratory test used to confirm the clinical diagnosis of Wilson's disease is normal. Are we up the creek in a canoe without a paddle? How is his mom going to take the bad news when I have built up her hopes so much? Why was I, just on clinical examination of the eyes, so sure that I knew Richard had a treatable disease?

Clinical Diagnosis is Always More Important than Any Test

Measurement of copper and copper proteins is a science, and a laboratory that does this determination should be thoroughly equipped to do it properly. Clinically, this patient has severe Wilson's disease, and yet the laboratory has reported a normal value for the blood protein usually deficient in the disease. What should we do about that? Which is correct: the laboratory value that says Richard doesn't have absent ceruloplasmin or my clinical diagnosis of Wilson's Disease? What would you do to resolve this dilemma? What is the more trustworthy evidence: the lab result or the clinical picture?

Reader, what would you do?

Answer: we should march down to the laboratory and talk with the technician who did the test to find out what's what.

Lab Director Migliori: "Bernie, what's up?"

Me: "I have a patient with Wilson's Disease, and your lab reported a normal value for ceruloplasmin. That has to be an error, so let's find out what happened."

Director Migliori and I march over to the tech who did the test.

"Let's see you repeat the test."

Re-examination of the same specimen under my supervision and that of the doctor in charge of the clinical laboratory showed no detectable ceruloplasmin. Zero! Richard has no ceruloplasmin in his blood. The clinical diagnosis is confirmed.

What Happened

When the technician did the test originally, she got a zero value also. She felt she had made an error in running the test and, therefore, she proceeded to enter a normal value in her report. As this case illustrates, absolute honesty and scientific integrity in the laboratory are vital to proper diagnosis of Wilson's Disease or any other disease. So, what should be done with the technician who reported a false laboratory result? What would you do, dear reader?

I pause for reply.

The technician was fired, of course.

A similar problem occurred with one of my patients from Mexico. He had severe systemic lupus erythematosus. The blood test usually positive in that condition is the anti-nuclear antibody. His test was reported back as normal. Repeat on the same specimen got a value in excess of 25,000. Normal is less than 20. This technician kept getting such high titers with each dilution of the specimen that he thought he was doing the test wrong, so he proceeded to report a normal value. He was fired.

Other Lab Results Confirm the Diagnosis

Richard's urine copper was sky high: 1,200 micrograms per 24 hours. Normal is less than 40. His urine copper excretion increased to 3,600 micrograms per 24 hours when I gave him the penicillamine. The penicillamine is an agent that binds copper and helps excrete copper in the urine. No normal person excretes that amount of copper after penicillamine, so the diagnosis of Wilson's Disease is amply confirmed, and the effectiveness of penicillamine as a treatment in Richard's case is proved.

I read 917 papers on Wilson's Disease published between 1966 and 1986 and could find no double-blind prospective controlled study comparing the effectiveness of actual treatment and placebo. Nevertheless, there is overwhelming consensus among neurologists that conventional treatments for Wilson's Disease are highly effective. Thus, if a treatment really works, you don't need statistical analysis or a big expensive clinical trial to prove it works. Many of the currently available medicines are only marginally effective because the test to prove they are effective involves only a statistical proof. Really effective treatments like L-DOPA for Parkinson's disease or penicillin for pneumonia needed no massive prospective randomized (and expensive) clinical trials to prove they work. Observing the effect on individual patients can be and should be evidence enough.

Because the fundamental problem in Wilson's Disease is excessive accumulation of copper in tissues, treatment should also consist in decreasing copper intake. Copper intake is decreased by administering a low copper diet. So, I educated mom about the copper content of foods and warned her to avoid those with the highest copper content like nuts, chocolate, coffee, and lobster.

"Sorry about lobster. Lobster blood is copper based, unlike human blood, which is iron based. So, no lobster for Richard."

Potassium iodide 20 milligrams four times daily binds copper and thereby decreases absorption by creating insoluble copper iodide, which is excreted in the stool. Zinc supplements induce metallothioneins that also decrease copper absorption.

Result

Richard's problems with blood, liver, kidney, and brain reversed or improved, and he returned to work. Mom was pleased as punch with the improvements. So was I. And yes, his brown eyes turned blue.

About trace metals: copper is essential to human health because it is a component of many essential enzyme systems, including cytochrome C oxidase, superoxide dismutase, tyrosinase, and dopamine beta-hydroxylase. But copper is toxic when present in above-normal amounts, as it is in Wilson's Disease.

Other essential metals are manganese, vanadium, iron, molybdenum, cobalt, zinc, and chromium. Each is at the center of an enzyme system, and each probably has a specific transport protein and a specific regulatory pathway for excretion in the bile. Knowing how human disease works its havocs, it is reasonable to conclude that there is at least one disease caused by the excess of each of these metals and one disease caused by a deficiency of each of these metals. The reason we don't know more about such diseases is that funds for basic research on them were cut off in the 1960s in order to pay for the trip to the moon. A similar problem is occurring now. Medical research funds are being cut, sometimes cut for silly reasons. Gun research is now a no-no. Research on sex, especially transgender and homosexual issues, is also a no-no. I am not making this up. Congress has specifically defunded research into these issues where certain groups do not want to know what's what. Even much-needed climate change research is now on the chopping block! Imagine what dodos the current mass of Republican politicians will look like 20 years from now when their ostrich-head-in-the-sand approach to human problems is exposed. In my opinion, republicans are very good at groupthink. Consequently, we will suffer.

The presence of a metallic ion in the center of an enzyme system is a consequence of the evolutionary history of life on this planet. Indeed, the first enzymes were the trace metals themselves, which are able to lower energy barriers, thereby facilitating electron transfer and chemical reactions. Subsequently, in the course of evolution, pyrrole groups were engrafted around trace elements, and last, proteins were attached to the pyrroles. Thus, it is no accident the usual enzyme structure consists of a metal surrounded by pyrroles and a protein.

Reference: Bernard M. Patten, Wilson's Disease, in *Parkinson's Disease and Movement Disorders*, edited by Joseph Jankovic and Eduardo Tolosa, Chapter 14, 179-190, Urban & Schwarzenberg, Baltimore-Munich, 1988.

Now let's go from the sublime to the ridiculous by discussing a woman who was speeding.

Tableau Twenty-Seven:

The Jewish Housewife Who Was Speeding

University Heights Hospital, Bronx

The job I got was through my friend and fellow resident, Don Palatucci. His father was an attending physician at a small hospital in the Bronx that needed physician coverage nights and weekends. In those days in New York, we were licensed to "practice medicine and surgery in the state of New York" the day we graduated from medical school. Thus, there was no problem with licensing. And there was little in the way of malpractice suits. My entire malpractice premium for the year was $100. The following year, I got a letter from the company apologizing for raising the premium to $125! When I retired from Baylor, my malpractice premium was $11,000, and I had a good record. Some neurosurgeons and some orthopedic surgeons were paying more than $100,000 a year in premiums! Some malpractice cases are justified, and most are not, as we shall see in the next section of this book.

Moonlighting at University Heights Hospital, Bronx, New York

The job was easy and paid nine dollars an hour. Usually, I sat in the doctor's on-call room on the 4th floor and read textbooks. When there were no more textbooks to read, I read novels. If you name a novel, any novel of any worth, chances are I read it during the time I was a house officer at the University Heights Hospital on Tremont Avenue in the Bronx.

$9 an Hour to Read Novels. Hot Dog!

Usually, there were no admissions. The most number of admissions I had in one night was three. Usually, the patients had simple illnesses easily handled, like a stroke, heart attack, congestive heart failure, atrial fibrillation, gastrointestinal bleeding, pneumonia, and so forth. These were conditions I could take care of in my sleep because of all the patients I took care of during internship at the New York Hospital Cornell Medical Center. There were a few emergency surgeries in the early morning hours that I assisted at. The surgeons were quite capable and did a fine job. They also let me close the wound. That was good experience.

The hospital also had an emergency room, which was seldom visited. And when people did drop in, the nurse usually sent them elsewhere rather than bother me. One night, the head nurse called me to come down to see a patient.

Nurse: "There's a Jewish housewife down here speeding. You had better come take care of her."

Me: "Tell her to go home and not take that stuff anymore."

271

Note: speeding is what happens when you take speed. Speed is slang for amphetamine, a stimulant that can temporarily reduce fatigue, increase mental activity, and give a feeling of wellbeing, but which also raises blood pressure and can cause headache if the blood pressure goes too high.

Nurse: "I can't measure her diastolic pressure, so it must be above 300. God only knows what her systolic pressure is. She might bleed into the coco (head). She has a headache—real bad."

Me: "I'll be right down."

The patient was a nice 28-year-old Jewish housewife with terrible teeth and terrible breath (common among speeders, I don't know why). She had taken too much speed and now had a gigantic problem with blood pressure and headache. I injected hydralazine 10 milligrams, which lowered the blood pressure to normal within 10 minutes. The pulse rate went way up as the blood pressure came down, but I was not concerned, as that was a known effect of the drug and should cause no problem. The Jewish housewife left the emergency room with a normal blood pressure and no headache.

The Jewish Housewife Saved My Life

Where is she? I wish I could find her and hug her and tell her how she saved my life. But alas, she is gone, and I don't know where to find her. Like the wandering Aengus, I may never find her and never pluck the golden apples of the sun, the silver apples of the moon. If I had not been called to see her, if she had not speeded that night, and if she had not come to the emergency room because of severe headache, chances are that night I would have met my death, and Tremont Avenue would have been a hot street of murder.

When I got back, the on-call room was a mess. Someone had shot up the room from across the street. The TV was smashed, and there were bullet holes all over the east wall at about the height of my chest. If I had been at the desk where I usually sat reading novels, the bullets would have hit me in the head and probably damaged the novel that I had been reading, which was *Middlemarch* by George Eliot—a masterpiece.

The Bronx was a dangerous place in those days and probably still is today. Most of us doctors carried guns. My gun was a Walther PPK 380 semiautomatic. I had a license to carry, and I got my license without much trouble. When I applied for my gun license, the precinct captain said, "Doc, to get a license to carry in New York City, you need the endorsement of four people who have a license to carry."

The Jewish Housewife Who Was Speeding

"What! I don't know anyone."

"Yes, you do. You're at Columbia, right."

He pulled out a sheet with the names of my professors and fellow residents at Columbia. The acting chief of medicine had a snub nose in his belt. The professor of ENT had a berretta in his ankle holster. The professor of neurosurgery had a Walther in his pocket. He suggested I get a Walther because it was so concealable. He said, "You really need a gun around here."

He was right. One time when I was headed up Tremont Avenue, the drug dealers were having a shoot-out on the street. Twice as I approached the hospital, I had to duck sniper bullets from the apartment across the street. In Casablanca, Rick (the Humphrey Bogart character) tells Major Strasser, the Nazi, "Major, there are some places in the Bronx even you wouldn't want to invade." That was a good line and good advice.

About the shot up on-call room. No sense calling the cops. They were afraid to get involved. One time, I asked two cops to chase the man who had stolen my wallet. The criminal disappeared into the apartment project across the street. "No way, Doc. We can't go in there. Too dangerous."

That night, the night of the speeding Jewish housewife, I slept under the bed. After that, the physician's bed was positioned away from the windows against the west wall, so that shots from across the street could not hit the bed.

One Last Patient

This is going to be a short one because I mentioned I would tell about another patient with a magnesium problem.

South Hampton Socialite

She entered the hospital in status epilepticus, a fatal condition where the patient has one major grand mal seizure after another without regaining consciousness in between. The usual treatments did not work, and she continued to seize for two days while I applied every treatment I could think of. We even did four vessel arteriograms to outline brain vessels, looking for tumors, abscess, subdural hematoma, etc. All normal. Day three, a Friday, the laboratory reported the serum magnesium 0.3 mEq/L, a very low value. Intravenous magnesium stopped the seizures within five minutes. Bingo! That was the Dx. She had major motor seizures because of magnesium deficiency, just the opposite of the other patient you were told about who had too much magnesium.

Now that the patient was awake and talking, I got a history. She drank at least 10 gin martinis a day! Alcohol does wash magnesium out in the urine, but this patient also had a unique kidney defect that caused her to excrete magnesium in the urine whether she was drinking or not. Therefore, she needed extra magnesium as a supplement to prevent the recurrence of seizures. She proved she needed the supplement on a second admission. She felt so normal, she stopped the magnesium and again entered the hospital in status epilepticus with a low serum magnesium. This time, she didn't have to seize for two days. The seizures stopped within minutes of administration of intravenous magnesium.

At medical grand rounds, I presented her case to Robert Loeb, distinguished visiting professor from Columbia University College of Physicians and Surgeons, who amazingly, right after hearing the history, got the diagnosis right off the bat. Did Tom Jones, our chief resident, tip him off? Must have.

I started the presentation by stating I too was from Columbia, but not distinguished. Everyone seemed to agree with that statement. Everyone also agreed the patient would have died had the magnesium deficiency not been discovered and treated.

Record Two:
Medical Malpractice (Med–Mal) and Trials of an Expert Witness

"Man is but a reed, the weakest thing in nature, but he is a thinking reed."

Blaise Pascal after having discovered the properties of the cycloid

In February 1824 on rounds at the Hotel-Dieu with Doctor Guillaume Dupuytren, the famous neurologist and professor, who loved Beef Wellington even though the dish was named after the general who defeated Napoleon at Waterloo in 1815, explained his notion that he can instantly detect hydrocephalus in a patient from the manner in which the patient carries his head.

Then seeing a patient in the distance, Dupuytren said to his students— "Do you see that man with his hand on his face and his head almost to his shoulder. Now take notice: the man has hydrocephalus."

The man was called up, and Dupuytren told him, "I know what ails you, but come, tell us about it yourself."

The patient replied he had a toothache.

"Take that," said Dupuytren, giving him a box on the ear.

The patient, annoyed and cowed by the big professor, retreated silently to the dental clinic.

Rounds continued as if nothing special had happened. Once again, the emperor had not been fully informed about the state of his new clothes.

Neurology Rounds with the Maverick

Samuel Goodrich, MD, American eyewitness

Harvard archive, Boston, 1824

As the above report shows, mistakes were made even by the world's great neurologists.

The purpose of record two is to show how the legal system impacted the practice of medicine in the golden age. My narrative tone is different from the nice Doctor Patten in record one because this is a fight between plaintiff and defendant. Sometimes the fight is brutal, but the resolution of disputes by the legal system, according to my attorney friend Lee Hamel, is better than guns.

Tableau Twenty-Eight:

Malpractice Cases against Me

Malpractice Case One

The first case against me occurred during internship. The first assignment I had was to the Hospital for Special Surgery, which was the part of the New York Hospital that handled rheumatic diseases and bone and orthopedic problems. The rotation there had only two house officers, myself, and Gwynn, the resident. We alternated call. Every other night and every other weekend would find me in the hospital taking care of patients. One of the duties of the medical resident and medical intern was to read the x-rays and to read the electrocardiograms. We also did the medical consultations when the surgeons wanted someone to give the medical OK, what they called medical clearance, for orthopedic surgery.

The patient who needed clearance was the wife of the vice president of General Motors. She was an old lady who had a bunch of people hanging around her room. They were at her beck and call and fetched her candies (for sure), flowers (definitely), booze (I think), and so forth. Most of these helpful people were black and received lavish tips in cash from the patient. That was a fact and not a racist remark. The woman was surrounded by a bunch of black hangers-on.

Her medical exam was good, and the chest x-ray and EKG were normal, so I saw no reason not to clear her for hip surgery. But I did write in the chart at the end of my clearance note: "This patient is obviously surrounded by an entourage of goldbrickers." And I signed my note in bright blue ink, my calling card signature, Bernard M. Patten, assistant physician.

She was unhappy with the surgical result, and her lawyers summoned the records. In those days, no orthopedic surgeon would testify against another orthopedic surgeon, and thus there was no case about the surgery. New York law required an expert witness to say that there had been negligence, and if you couldn't get an expert to do that, you didn't get to first base in a malpractice case. Texas law runs that way now, but in the old days, it was quite different, as you will soon see when I tell you about my malpractice cases in Texas.

Anyway, she wanted to work out her anger on someone, so she told her lawyers to sue me for defamation of character. Her entire case rested on the medical record wherein there appeared in my distinctive handwriting the statement that she was surrounded by goldbrickers. The only defense was to prove the statement true.

The judge eventually ruled in the woman's favor and let the case go to trial on the issue. He said that although I had written goldbricker, what I actually meant was gold digger. A goldbricker is a swindler. The judge sensed that I meant gold digger, which, I guess, is what I meant. Looking back on the situation, the judge was correct. I really meant to call them gold diggers, but in my ignorance, I wrote the wrong word.

Physicians, nurses, and technicians who had come in contact with the patient and her entourage testified that yes, she was surrounded by an entourage of goldbrickers and gold diggers! Much to the poor woman's embarrassment, the judge wouldn't let the case go to the jury. Instead, he said that the truth had been proven. The statement was correct, and therefore, the defense must win. The judge dismissed the case with prejudice. That meant they could not come against me again.

Lesson: There is an old Irish slogan: "Never write what you can say, and never say what you can wink." Be careful about what you write, even if it is the truth.

Malpractice Case Two

The next case troubled my sleep for years. The reason this case bothered me was that it was about medical malpractice, called med-mal by the legal profession, and not about defamation of character, which was the cause of the previous suit. My overinflated, gigantic ego was damaged by the suit because a med-mal made it seem like I was a bad doctor.

The patient was a woman in her twenties who was wheelchair bound due to weakness of her legs. The neurological evaluation showed that she had a peripheral neuropathy, and I did a nerve biopsy as part of the attempt to find the cause of the nerve disease. The scene in the operating room is still crystal clear in my mind because it was the first and the only time that we had seen real dirt on a patient's leg prior to the operation. It was caked-on mud, and then and there I should have canceled the biopsy. Instead, the O.R. nurses went to work cleaning the area with soap and hot water, and after that, the area was painted with betadine to sterilize the skin over the nerve.

The biopsy site got infected. Miss Lopez sued me for $300,000 because of the infection.

The actual lawsuit made me look negligent. It said I did not care for the infection, that I did not prescribe an antibiotic, and that the infection continued to rage long after the patient left the hospital. All that was not true. I personally visited the patient. I personally cleaned the wound. I personally changed the dressings each day. I did prescribe an antibiotic, and the infection cleared up, and the patient left the hospital infection free. That her lawyer could say such things about me was absurd. Obviously, he had not read the medical record. But even more absurd was the fact that this patient was suing me. She had gotten an excellent response to the treatment, correction of a vitamin deficiency, had been restored to normal, and was working full-time as a nurse. Despite the facts that were on my side, I still could not shake the idea that I was being sued, and that someone had put into writing that I was a terrible doctor. My ego and my reputation were under attack, and I took it all personally. Ethel was also adversely affected by the lawsuit because I sometimes woke up screaming and in a cold sweat from a bad dream centered around this caper.

My lawyer was no help. He is now very famous, and I could not possibly hire him to defend me because I could not possibly pay his fee. He has a special moniker here in Houston, which would be immediately recognized by the old-timers in this fair city. Let's call him "Racehorse."

Me: "Racehorse, how's my case going?"

Racehorse: "Jesus, I told you: don't bother me. I will take care of everything."

Me: "Sorry, Racehorse, it is just bugging me. I am having trouble sleeping and thinking about what might happen. This whole thing is interfering with my work, my sleep, my digestion, my marriage, my life."

Racehorse: "She is going to make a very good witness—a very good witness for us! For us! Did you hear me! So, forget it! When we go to trial, I will take her apart. Meanwhile, don't bother me. I'm busy. I have much more important cases to deal with than your little piece of shit."

Years went by, and my case finally came up.

Racehorse: "Miss Lopez, what do you think of Doctor Patten?"

She: "Oh, I love him. I think he is a great doctor."

Racehorse: "OK, Miss Lopez. Let's get this straight. You like Doctor Patten. Is that correct?"

She: "No. I told you, I love him. He is a great doctor."

Racehorse: "Did Doctor Patten do anything to help you?"

She: "He cured me."

Racehorse: "Miss Lopez, I am trying to understand. You say he helped you. Is that right?"

She: "No, I said he cured me. I was in a wheelchair. I couldn't walk. I couldn't work. Look at me. I am back to normal. I am working full time."

Racehorse: "OK. Miss Lopez. You love Doctor Patten, and you think he helped you. Is that right?"

She: "He cured me! I told you. Why do you keep changing what I say?"

Racehorse: "One more question, Miss Lopez."

Guadalupe Lopez sits there waiting; nods her head but says nothing. She does look good, much better than before my treatment. And she does seem grateful for her recovery. But on the other hand, she did have an infection. It was trivial but real, so maybe she deserves some sort of compensation. But certainly not $300,000. On the other hand, she signed the consent form before operation, and that did mention infection as a possible side effect and complication of surgery. And she is a nurse, so she had to know some wounds get infected. What do you think? Should she win her case or not?

I pause for reply.

Racehorse Continues with One Last Question

Racehorse: "OK, Miss Lopez. Let's get this straight. You love Doctor Patten, and you think he cured you. Then, why are you suing him?"

She: "That's easy. I met my lawyer, Mr. Rivera here (she nods at Rivera), at a cocktail party, and he said I would get some money from the infection and that it wouldn't hurt Doctor Patten because Doctor Patten is insured."

Bang! Bang! Bang!

Judge: "Young Lady, you should be ashamed of yourself. Case dismissed."

> **Lesson:** Don't forget that in real life there actually are simple people.

> **Lesson:** Follow your lawyer's advice, and don't let your fears get the best of you.

Whoa! Talking about simple people reminds me of my friend Fred whose med-mal case never got off the ground. Fred did a vasectomy and told the couple they could not get pregnant. The wife got pregnant, and she and her husband accused Fred of doing a poor job. Fred reopened and found he had done things right. It turned out the wife took Fred's advice too literally and didn't realize she could get pregnant if she had sex with another man, not her husband.

The next med-mal hit me less emotionally. Suffering produces wisdom. The anti-climax of the Lopez case taught me a lesson. The wisdom derived from my first malpractice case is that I worried too much and too long about what came to nothing.

Malpractice Case Three

In this case, the patient was a young woman with severe migraine headaches who told me that if she continued to have headaches, she was going to kill herself. Because none of the usual treatments worked, I thought I might try Sansert. Sansert is usually effective, but it does have a serious side effect. It can cause fibrous connective tissue to grow in the retroperitoneal area. Sometimes, the growth of such tissue obstructs the drainage of urine from the kidney. The pressure on the kidney causes impaired kidney function and dilation of the kidney pelvis, a condition called hydronephrosis.

Sansert produced immediate relief of headache, but when the Sansert was stopped, the headache returned just as severe as before. To prevent the side effect, the usual procedure is to alternate three months on Sansert and one month off. The month off was the problem because during that time, the patient would have to suffer and try not to kill herself. Although the patient was told to stop the Sansert for the required month, it may be that she did not stop it. Or if she did stop it, she stopped it for only one day because she couldn't stand the headache. In fact, on one visit, she did tell me that she tried to stop but restarted within a day because the headaches were so severe. Considering what she was suffering, no one could blame her. But that is the way to trouble. That is the way to obstruct urinary drainage and cause hydronephrosis.

She did develop the hydronephrosis, and she sued. Among the many terrible things said about me was the crux of the complaint:

"Doctor Patten negligently did not warn the patient about the possibility of the well-known side effect connected with Sansert."

The chart, however, had a written note in my hand saying I did warn her, and, miracle of miracles, my nurse, Dale Salazar, put in the chart she had discussed that specific side effect with the patient. And, miracles of miracles, Dale had the patient read the Sansert package insert with the warning on it and sign the package insert that she had read the warning. Dale then pasted the signed package insert with the patient's statement and signature into the chart.

Conclusion: the patient's lawyer had filed the lawsuit before he read the chart! It is also possible that the patient told him wrong because she did not remember the warnings, and he assumed she knew what she was talking about.

My attorney, John Raley of the firm of Fulbright & Jaworski, made much of that. All the written evidence supported the idea that the patient had been warned, and the written evidence contradicted the major claim of the lawsuit.

The lawsuit was withdrawn, only to reappear weeks later in modified form. Now the suit said:

"Doctor Patten did discuss the side effect, and the patient did read the package insert and the warning. But Doctor Patten, with total disregard of the patient's health, took the patient aside in his clinic office and told her to forget those things because the side effect would never happen to her."

After the second filing, my lawyer, John, asked me:

"Well, what the hell did you actually tell her?"

"John, for the life of me, I can't remember talking about the fibrosis or the other side effects, but I think I may have told her the side effect of hydronephrosis was extremely rare, and it was probably not going to affect her."

John: "If I were your patient, your statement would have meant I didn't have anything to worry about. Don't you think?"

Malpractice Cases against Me

Me: "I wanted her to take the Sansert because it was a matter of life or death. She really meant it about suicide. If the headaches continued, she said she would kill herself. I believed her."

John: "I'll get you off the hook."

About John Raley: he was the best lawyer for me. Perfect really. He was upbeat, optimistic, happy, smart, and confided in me about his private life and private problems. He was a lawyer who took care of me not as a stranger, but as a friend. John and I would meet at his office, discuss the case for maybe seven minutes, and then spend the rest of the time dueling to see who could recite the most Shakespeare. At noon, we went to lunch and then went back to the office to continue the duel. For him, I am sure, these were billable hours. For both of us, these were hours of fun, a lot of them. John was the only person I have ever known who knew, by heart, as much Shakespeare as I do.

John got me off the hook. He pointed out how the story had changed to suit the convenience of the plaintiffs.

The judge said to the plaintiff's attorney, "Next time, get your story straight the first time around." Bang! "Case dismissed."

And that was that. This next med-mal was even more stupid, but the patient's illness fascinated me.

Malpractice Case Four: the Smoker with Chronic Obstructive Pulmonary Disease

The patient was a 28-year-old man who smoked seven packs of Salem cigarettes a day for at least seven years. Yes, I said seven packs of Salems a day. Seven packs a day is even more than John Wayne, who was a five-pack-a-day man. P.S. Wayne died of a combination of lung cancer and stomach cancer.

> **Lesson:** Don't smoke. Burning tobacco has over 70 known chemicals that cause cancer.

My patient would wake, throw his legs over the edge of the bed, reach for the pack, light up, burn one, inhaling deeply, and then get out of bed. He smoked when he shaved, he smoked when he ate, and he smoked while he did it with his wife.

On exam, he was weak and fatigued easily, had tremors of his fingers and toes. When he walked, he was unsteady, and he got short of breath just crossing the room. Electromyogram was normal, and the muscle biopsy showed mild neurogenic atrophy.

This kind of illness was well reported in the old medical literature when people chewed green tobacco, which had a much higher content of nicotine than cured tobacco. In each case, there was unexplained neuromuscular disease with weakness and easy fatiguability, sometimes associated with shortness of breath, palpitations, tremors, and muscle wasting. Electromyograms are usually normal, but some patients have had slowed nerve conduction times. Complete remission occurs when tobacco consumption stops. The recovery is biphasic. The condition rapidly improves within a week of stopping the tobacco. Then there is further slower improvement as the victim gains weight and muscle bulk.

In addition to causing muscle disease, chronic nicotine poisoning can cause a grave myasthenic syndrome, especially among those who chew tobacco during their entire waking hours. Green tobacco poisoning in people picking tobacco after a rainfall is due to the absorption of nicotine through the skin. The pickers collapsed in the field and had to be carried home.

As chief of nerve and muscle disease division at Baylor, the cases of nicotine poisoning usually crossed my path. I had a collection of cases including an 11-year-old girl who smoked two packs a day (Salem again) for over two years and a 46-year-old man who was so addicted to tobacco he used to stash and hide it around the house. That man even invented a way of administering nicotine to himself during sleep. He put tobacco in a child's milk bottle and added water, shook the stuff to put some nicotine into solution, and then sucked the nipple as he slept. That man, an attorney, was able to stop tobacco, and he felt "better than in years." His grip strength improved 33% within three months of stopping the tobacco.

Indeed, the neuromuscular effects of nicotine have found application in game management, where hundreds of animals have been immobilized, captured, and translocated after nicotine administration by a dart gun. Within three minutes, animals hit by a nicotine-bearing dart develop locomotor ataxia (unsteady gait) and a flaccid paralysis. Recovery occurs within three hours. Acute nicotine toxicity often occurs either from accidental ingestion of nicotine-containing insecticides or after oral or rectal administration of tobacco. And yes, I personally have removed a pack of Camel cigarettes from the rectum of a patient in coma. How that pack got there and why we'll never know because he died. His death may have followed and been due to seizures. Large amounts of nicotine administered by rectum can cause convulsions and sometimes death.

> **Lesson:** Putting cigarettes up your rectum is not a good idea! Don't do it.

At the end of World War II, a trio of Frenchmen decided to celebrate by drinking brandy. One of the men reached up on a shelf and pulled down a bottle of a dark brown liquid. They drank a toast, "Finnie la guerre!" Too bad the dark liquid they ingested was not brandy. It was nicotine insecticide. All three agreed that the drink tasted funny. Then all three had major motor seizures and died.

> **Lesson:** Don't store your insecticides next to your booze.

For a time, my 28-year-old patient reduced his dose of Salems to two packs a day. His muscle disease improved, but the shortness of breath did not. He couldn't stay away from the bigger doses and went back to his seven packs per day. His chronic obstructive pulmonary disease worsened, and he died.

For the life of me, I couldn't figure out how to help him. The smoking had to stop. But stopping it didn't seem possible, despite the clear warnings about what would happen if he continued to smoke. This patient was truly addicted to the great god nicotine. Have you any ideas of how this patient could have been better cared for? If so, let me know. There is no question that my medical care in his case was completely ineffective. Maladaptive behavior, be it expressed as alcoholism, cigarette addiction, obesity, excessive TV watching, obsessive work, or lack of joy in life is not easily ameliorated, much less abolished. The ridiculousness of human behavior and the curious sadness that underlies much of it is the root cause of Molière's hilarious comedies.

My patient's widow sued me on the grounds I had not been forceful enough in warning that if he continued to smoke, he would soon be dead. The wheels fell off that argument when the court read my notes. *Res ipse loquitur* = legalese for the case is blindly obvious. (Literally: "The thing speaks for itself.") Everybody knows or should know smoking is bad for the lungs. No special medical warning is needed. Case dismissed.

Notice by the time of the last case I had a complete trust in the legal system. The more you learn, the less you fear. Learn not in the sense of academic study but in the practical understanding of life. Does that make sense?

Nicotine is Toxic

In view of the evidence, nicotine toxicity should be considered in all tobacco users who have unexplained weakness. Because the final proof of the diagnosis of tobacco-induced neuromuscular disease depends on the demonstration of remission or significant improvement after the tobacco stopped, it is a good idea to get baseline measurements of body weight, muscle size, head and leg holding times, and grip strength before asking the victim to abstain from tobacco use. Failure to improve after tobacco is discontinued does not exclude the diagnosis because, especially in cases of long-term exposure, permanent damage to the nervous system may have already occurred. It is likely that high school ballplayers who chew tobacco are functioning under a nicotine-induced handicap. That has to be the case because science is always right.

Nicotine in history

When, on the 29th of October 1492, Christopher Columbus cast anchor off the shores of Cuba, he met native men and women who held in their hands cylindrical objects made of a dry leaf, one end of which was aflame and from the other end of which they inhaled smoke. These cylinders, called tobaccos, were simply the ancestors of our modern cigars and cigarettes. From these humble beginnings, because of psychosocial motives reinforced by the pharmacological effects of nicotine, which almost inevitably cause dependence, and in some rare cases addiction, tobacco has made a conquest of the world, probably for all time.

In the future, tobacco toxicity will be decreased by more effective control of some toxic components such as tar, toxic trace elements, and carbon monoxide, but a method to eliminate nicotine toxicity is out of the question, for without nicotine people would be as likely to use tobacco as they would be to blow bubbles, light sparklers, or chew gum. It is the nicotine content of tobacco, as one cigarette company booklet from the first New York World's Fair so aptly states, that makes "tobacco the solace of a troubled world."

Last Med-Mal Case, This One Not against Me

Preston Harrison was sued by a family that suffered the loss of their loved one. The patient was a young father who fell off a roof because he had a grand-mal seizure. Preston did all the appropriate tests, including scans and examination of spinal fluid. The results were negative. The major consideration in the case was, of course, brain tumor. Adult-onset seizures are often caused by a brain tumor. Sure enough, eventually, the tumor showed on the scans, and eventually the patient died. Preston was accused of neglecting the patient and failing to diagnose the tumor in time for a cure.

The plaintiffs had a neurologist expert who testified that the tumor would have been curable if it had been diagnosed in time and that he himself had personally taken care of and cured over 800 patients with that kind of tumor. The neurologist was well known to me because he had been on the faculty of the Department of Neurology when I was trying to administer the department. His name shall remain secret because of the black marks on his soul. Let's call him Henry Mushroom. I fired him because he was a lazy son-of-a-bitch who didn't show up on multiple occasions to round with the residents at the VA Hospital. In fact, there was little evidence that Henry ever did any useful work.

The brain tumor in question was a glioblastoma multiforme, the most malignant brain tumor you can get and the one that killed Senator Ted Kennedy and the same tumor that killed another Senator (John McCain) who had run for president. I could not find a single report in the world's medical literature of any patient who had ever survived such a tumor. The great neurosurgeon, Harvey Cushing, had assembled about 800 cases and reported all patients had died. Thus, my testimony contradicted Henry Mushroom's. I claimed that Preston had done everything right and the problem was not with medical care but with the extremely malignant nature of the tumor itself. The fault was with the disease and not the doctor. I also claimed that Doctor Mushroom had not taken care of over 800 patients with glioblastoma multiforme and had probably not cured any. And furthermore, if he had witnessed a cure, he should have written a paper reporting the event. I also claimed that earlier detection of the tumor would not have made a difference in the eventual outcome. The patient would have died, no matter what.

Plaintiff's Lawyer: "Doctor Patten, are you calling Doctor Henry Mushroom a liar?"

Me: "Yes. I am." (For some reason the lawyer seemed shocked by my direct answer to his stupid question. After a long pause, he changed the subject.)

Plaintiff's Lawyer: "Are you sure that early detection of the tumor would not have given the patient a chance, even a small chance of cure?"

Me: "It is theoretically possible that very early detection might have given the patient a chance. But the preponderant weight of evidence would be against that possibility." (Notice how I have learned how to speak legalese. Civil cases require that the preponderant weight of evidence come in on the winning side. Thus 51% versus 49% would tip the result in Preston's favor.)

Plaintiff's Lawyer: "Doctor Patten, one last question. How often do you think a CAT scan should have been done to detect the tumor at the earliest possible time?"

Me: "Every 15 minutes." The lawyer scowled. The jury laughed. The judge banged and demanded order.

Poor Preston. He was literally shaken up by this case, and he was shaking so much he couldn't walk and had to be carried out of the courtroom. We went to lunch at a local restaurant that served chicken fried steak. It was smothered in some kind of white gravy, and I ate very little. The white gravy looked good and smelled good but was too salty and seemed to burn my tongue. I never use salt on my food, so I am not used to even a little salt.

Preston was too upset to eat or drink anything. He also was unable to talk, literally speechless. No kidding. That's how bad we physicians regard a med-mal. Naturally, I was sympathetic because I had been through a similar kind of excessive worry with my first med-mal. But now I was an experienced pro with full faith and confidence in the legal system.

Recess is over. We are back. But the jury is nowhere in sight.

Preston's lawyer: "The judge instructed the jury, and the jury is out to reach a verdict. Don't expect too much. This is Daingerfield, Texas, where they have a unique legal system designed to transfer money from outside Daingerfield to the locals."

After 17 minutes, the jury returns. The vote is 12 to 0 in Preston's favor, and that was naturally the end of that. I tell the story for what it is worth.

While we are touching on the subject of glioblastoma, I would like to mention a personal experience. In 1988, I made a will. My secretary, Mary Anne, was one witness, and my resident was the other witness. When the resident signed, he made a strange remark: "I have a feeling that you will live longer than me."

Me: "George, don't talk that way. It may tempt the gods."

Two weeks later, George was waiting at my office when I arrived at work.

George: "I have a brain tumor."

Me: "What? What makes you say that?"

George: "Yesterday, I arrived on my street but couldn't figure out which way to turn to get into my driveway, right or left."

Me: "Holy cow! The lesion is in the right hemisphere. This is serious."

The scan showed a highly malignant glioblastoma, which was exerting pressure on the brain and had already shifted midline structures from right to left. Surgery was scheduled for the following morning, but George didn't even make it to the O.R. While waiting to be wheeled in, he suddenly clutched his head and died. Autopsy showed a massive hemorrhage into the tumor had caused his death.

About Lawsuits

By age 55, nearly half of physicians have been sued for malpractice. General surgeons and obstetricians face the most risk. 64% of OB-GYN and 63% of surgeons were sued at least once during their careers, while only 16% of psychiatrists and 18% of pediatricians faced suits. Male doctors are more likely to be sued than female (40% versus 23%). The average expense in a lawsuit, according to the American Medical Association, was $54,165 according to data from 90,473 claims that closed between 2006 and 2015. Most claims are dropped or withdrawn or dismissed, but the average cost of defense for those suits is still high at $30,475, and that does not count money lost during downtime for the doctor. Only 7% of cases were decided by trial, and 88% of those trials came in for the doctor.

Conclusion: the malpractice game does take a toll on the healthcare system when the nation is trying to reduce health care costs. But the legal system, as my lawyer friend Lee Hamel told me, is "better than guns."

Trials of an Expert Witness

As a doctor seasoned by many confrontations with the legal system, I found that I became significantly less anxious about testifying in front of a judge and jury. When opposing counsel is contentious or argumentative during questioning, I am dramatically less bothered and keep my cool. One attorney friend explained that the legal system was "a dice game." Sometimes you win, and sometimes you don't. Some of the cases I testified as an expert witness for came out wrong and some came out right, proving that my lawyer friend was right. In many trials, the outcome is not predictable and seems significantly controlled by chance. Consider the following reports and see if you agree.

Case One: The Man Who Suffered an Exacerbation of His Chronic Multiple Sclerosis After a Trivial Fender Bender

The question at issue was whether a trivial stress could cause worsening of multiple sclerosis or not. Three neurologists testified it could, and they gave it for their opinion it did in this case, even though all agreed no physical trauma occurred, and the only possible stress was mental. I testified the opposite: that the accident had nothing to do with the worsening of the multiple sclerosis and tried to introduce into evidence several papers from Neurology, the official journal of the American Academy of Neurology, supporting my view. The judge would not allow the papers. She did allow me to state my opinion to the jury based on my experience and expertise.

Opposition counsel then asked, "Doctor Patten, how much were you paid to appear in court today?" I stated my usual fee, "$10,000." Then counsel asked me to tell the jury my total taxable income last year. Whoa! "Your Honor, I don't want to tell my income, and I don't see how it has any bearing on this case or my testimony." The judge, a very nice woman with gray hair and a good smile, said, "I am afraid you must answer the question, Doctor Patten."

I turned to the jury and announced in a loud voice, "Last year, my total taxable income was a little over $1,860,000, none of which came from testifying. Last year, I paid a little over $660,000 in federal income tax.

The jury came in for the defense. The exit poll showed that the jury thought my testimony was more believable than that of the other neurologists. They felt that someone with my kind of income was not testifying for the money. The lesson here is the lesson most lawyers already know: never ask a question if you don't, in advance, know the answer.

Two Other Cases Bothered My Sleep

One was a middle-aged biker that claimed he was paralyzed after an auto accident. I testified that he was normal on examination and was pretending to be ill. His laboratory tests, including the usual scans (auditory, visual, and somatosensory, evoked responses, and so forth) were all normal. And, as a matter of fact, the usual neurological tests for malingering were all positive. So, we had massive evidence that the guy was normal and massive evidence that he was pretending to be sick. Furthermore, the week before trial, the defense team had filmed the plaintiff skipping out his front door, jumping over a picket fence in front of his home, and then driving away on his motorcycle. The movie made him look very normal indeed and supported my idea this guy was a phony. Despite all that evidence, the jury awarded $4 million.

I told the insurance company lawyer, "Jesus, I am so sorry. I should have done a better job."

The reply was, "You did a great job, Doc. They were seeking 16 million. You saved us plenty of dough."

The next case was similar. A young woman with breast implants claimed the implants had caused her to be unable to walk. She was, according to my examination and the laboratory tests, completely normal. My testimony, in no uncertain terms, was that she was pretending to be sick so she could collect money from the implant companies. She was a malingerer. The opposing attorney pointed to the woman, who had that day come to court in a wheelchair and was slumped over, and said, "If she is so normal, Doctor, how come she looks so bad. How come she is in a wheelchair?"

My reply was, "She is probably having a very bad day." That elicited lots of laughs from the jury. But they still awarded $2 million. The insurance company lawyer told me, "What did you expect, Doc? This is California."

One Last Phony

This was a woman who was hit from behind by a teenage driver who admitted he was at fault. The only question before the court was the question of damages. The woman claimed she was significantly damaged and in severe pain. She came into court limping in such a way that I knew she was a phony. The plaintiff's lawyer asked, "Is there any member of this jury panel who had the privilege of going to medical school?" Of course, I raised my hand and was immediately excused. The next day, the plaintiff's lawyer asked me to have lunch with him. He said, "The reason I threw you off the panel is I knew you would know my client was a phony." I nodded in agreement. "As it was, we got $36,000 out of a case that was complete bullshit."

Record Three:
Breast Implants—How You Can Be Tough without a Gun

"I believe that companies deserve full credit for lying, cheating, and endangering people's health."

David Egilman, Brown University

Science, VOL 363, issue 6,425, p.337

"The one thing necessary, in life as in art, is to tell the truth."

Leo Nikolayevich Tolstoy (1828–1910)

Tableau Thirty:

The Breast Implant Adventure— the Beginning

For a long time, I used to ride to work in a limousine.

My first driver was Howard. He wasn't a good driver. He was a great driver. Always professional and efficient and always on time. Howard always looked like a concert pianist in black suit and tie ready to go on stage. They didn't scare Howard. But Howard had a big problem—chronic obstructive pulmonary disease. Even on nasal oxygen, he was falling asleep at the wheel.

My second driver was Trent, Howard's son. Trent was young and energetic and had a good smile. He was sometimes on time and sometimes not. He always dressed casually and sometimes even arrived in jeans. They did scare Trent. But Trent needed a job and Howard encouraged him to give it a try to see if he liked the job and to see if the job liked him.

One day, the limo ran out of gas on the Gulf Freeway (Interstate highway 45). That did not bother me because I just continued working while Trent called someone to get gas. On the road again, Trent said he was sorry he had not gassed the limo.

Me: "That's OK, Trent. You proved once again that without gas, the internal combustion engine won't work, and consequently, the limo won't go."

Trent: "Doctor Patten, I was thinking that I might come see you as a patient, so you can tell me if I have Adult Attention Deficit Disorder."

Me: "Forget it. You're just a discombobulant like so many young people these days."

Two weeks later, Trent was a new man. He was on time, organized, gassed the limo as he should, paid attention to the traffic on raceway 45 so that there were far fewer horns beeping at us, and so forth. He was so different, I had to ask.

Me: "Trent, what happened to you? You're a new man."

Trent: "I consulted another neurologist. He said I had Adult Attention Deficit Disorder, put me on some medicine, and changed my life."

Besides driving the limo, Trent did other work for me, including setting up my totem pole—that was before the murder, which I told about in my personal memoir "*The Wonderful World of Bernies*." Trent also ran messages and dealt with customs authorities who thought we might have smuggled drugs in the totem pole. He did not do my shopping. I had two women who shopped. They did an excellent job, and my family was always full of praise for the gifts they got at Christmas and for their birthdays. That's normal for busy doctors in the old days. The doctors had no time to shop or to do anything more than take care of patients. So, they hired experts to shop for them.

Ethel, my wife, learned my secret, but most family members thought that I, and not my shoppers, did the selections. OK, full disclosure: we also had multiple gardeners, a lawn service, a housekeeper, a pool woman, maids, and even a boatman. The boatman's job was to clean the boat each week and make sure it was in good running order. The boatman, Grant Graytok, was also to be on call 24/7 to rescue me and my friends in the event that there was a breakdown on the open water, a service that came in handy on several occasions I ran aground because I am a lousy sea captain.

In view of the large number of people I had doing things for me, Ethel thought next I would hire someone to service her. No way! Some jobs I reserve for myself.

My third driver was Linda, Howard's wife and Trent's mother. She was blond and beautiful and tough—no-nonsense woman. She carried a 32 snub nose detective special revolver to prove it. Yes, you guessed it: nothing scared Linda. So, Linda took over after the thugs beat the shit out of Trent.

Assault of Trent

One evening, after he had dropped me off, Trent was going home himself. While exiting the subdivision, Trent stopped to help a woman waving in distress. When Trent got out of the limo, four big guys jumped out of the woman's car and proceeded to kick the shit out of Trent. Trent had two broken ribs, multiple bruises, torn clothes, and a blackened right eye. The assailants fled before taking Trent's watch or wallet. At the time, we didn't know why they didn't steal anything.

Poor Trent. He lost his sang-froid. Trent learned the hard way this is a mean hard world. If you don't believe me, try walking around Houston or any big American city without a dime in your pocket.

Lesson: This is a mean hard world.

After his lesson in meanness, Trent refused to drive. Too dangerous! Reality was getting dense for him, too dense. He was still supercharged with the lingering angst of having survived real danger and having been beaten to a pulp. I don't blame Trent. His reluctance was within the normal range of human behavior. The normal thing after that kind of traumatic experience is to be scared.

But I told him, "Trent, no guts, no glory. Here's your chance to emerge a hero by facing down real BAD GUYS."

Still no.

Trent probably did the right thing because things soon got worse.

Breast Implant Adventure— the Middle

As I said, Linda, Trent's no-nonsense mother, took over. She had guts. Linda said, "I don't take no shit from nobody."

Hot dog! She was the kind of driver I needed. In my view, it was highly likely that Linda was hoping the hoods would try something on her so she could get revenge for what they had done to Trent.

It's Not Every Day That Your Nurse's House Burns Down

Three weeks later, September 14, 1994, in Alvin, Texas, at 2:45 a.m., Dale Salazar's home (Dale was my head clinical nurse) burned down. Dale, her husband, and six children (she's Hispanic) were not at home at the time. They were visiting relatives in Monterrey, Nuevo Leon, Mexico. The fire inspectors said that someone had committed arson. They could tell by the ignition sequence (everything went up at once—the fire didn't start in one place and spread) and by the things that melted, metals, mainly, especially vanadium and chromium, indicating higher temperatures occurred than expected in a natural accidental blaze. Foremost Insurance (yes, that's the name of Dale's insurance company) paid for the total loss $115,186. The thugs who had set the fire were never caught.

Some economic, social, political, scientific, and legal aspects of the breast implant research will be covered shortly. Here we continue the story of the criminal attacks related to medical research. Please don't feel sorry for me or Britta or Mavis or Glenn or Dale or Joanne or Cora any of the others who worked on this project. We were just doing our job and, most of the time, we liked the attention, the adventure, and the idea that some people thought enough about us and our research to attack us mercilessly. This hubris is in the Patten family tradition. Pop (my father) was a district attorney who sent many to jail and some to the electric chair. We had a tape recorder at home. If a death threat came in over the phone, it was recorded. When Pop got home, he drank a scotch and nodded for the tapes. "When I get out, Patten, I am going to get you and your family, etc." Usually, Pop smiled and said, "Shows I'm doing a good job! Pass the potatoes."

Please don't misinterpret my attempts to describe the foibles of human behavior as they affected our research as bitterness. That is a giant mistake made by some patients and by some of the patient advocacy groups. My aim is merely to capture the passion with which Britta and I, the aforementioned people on my office and clinic staff, and our colleagues pursued our adventure and our work. We were in it for knowledge and for the fun and for the adventure and to help people if we could.

Death Threats

On April 4, 1995, a decapitated rabbit arrived at home on our back-door mat. The rabbit's head was nowhere in sight. Its neck still gushed crimson red blood. Someone got confused. Easter was still a few weeks away. The rabbit arrived too early.

It reminded Ethel of the scene from the Godfather where the horse's head appears in the bed. Ethel said, "Someone is trying to tell you something."

My two cats, P.J. Patten and General Patten (the Tom) sniffed the dead rabbit and, overjoyed, started to eat. In their own perverted cat brains, in their feline imaginations, it appeared they thought I had given them still another token of my deep abiding affection. Or perhaps the cats thought this fresh-killed rabbit was part of a new service for cats sponsored by some new commercial organization that delivers for cats the way Pizza Hut delivers for humans.

But that was it—the moment I had stepped through the looking glass. After the decapitated animal arrived, I never felt entirely safe. Would you?

Criminals Break into the Muscle and Nerve Laboratory at the Baylor College of Medicine

On April 11, 1995, my technicians found, when they got to work, that my laboratory had been raided. They recoiled at the mess, slides removed and tossed about, reports gone over, and furniture overturned. On the bench where we usually receive the biopsy specimens, someone had placed a pair of crutches and some duct tape (see photo). That was nice, but my knee, injured in October 1994, had fully recovered. At the time, I didn't need crutches.

Two hours later, when I arrived at my academic office, I discovered that the papers I had left on my desk had disappeared. Those papers, about 200 pages of my research on the complications of breast implants, constituted my latest contribution to the scientific understanding of the subject. Don't worry. I learned my lesson from my patient, who was the environmental officer at that plant in Beaumont. In fact, there were copies distributed in different places to different people. I also had a copy at home.

That afternoon, I got a call from the brain scan laboratory. "We hope you are happy with all the copies of the brain scans on implanted women that we made yesterday for your fellow, Glenn."

"Glenn copied scans? That's impossible. Glenn has been out sick all week."

"Glenn was here, or, ugh, someone claiming he was Glenn was here, and we gave him the scans."

Thus, someone pretended they were Glenn and illegally got copies of those scans.

What does it all mean? Why would someone steal research data? What evil lurks in the hearts of men? The shadow knows, and so do I. Some person or persons is deeply interested in hiding the truth about implants. I wonder who? Commercial interests tend to ignore relevant data and push back. The real question now was: when will the war begin? I didn't have to wait long.

Houston Police Conduct an Investigation

Houston police said a professional did the job because they found no fingerprints either on the crutches or on the duct tape. To this day, the crime remains unsolved. We don't know how the criminals got the locked laboratory door opened or how they got past the Methodist Hospital security people posted by the elevators.

Perhaps these events relate to and can be understood in the context of the five to 10 calls to my home where the caller doesn't talk when I answer or when Ethel answers. When we say hello, the caller hangs up. At least, these anonymous callers were not trying to sell me another Visa Gold Card or ask for a donation.

Oh, yes, I almost forgot. Those folders from Forest Lawn Cemetery arrived each day. Thursdays, I usually got two. Then there were the anonymous letters that run like this: "Doctor Patten, social security only pays $225 for your funeral. You are responsible for the rest. Better prepare." Whoever wrote that note remains misinformed. They forgot that since I am a veteran, I get my very own bugler to play taps, and I get a free American flag, and a free funeral. I don't worry about paying for my funeral. The United States Government will pay for it if they find my body.

Killing Would Not Help

I wish I could have told the criminals killing me won't help. It was too late. There were seven papers in the press about the complications of breast implants. No stopping them! The damage they will do is prefixed like a V2 rocket headed to London after flame out. It will continue on course governed only by Newtonian laws of motion as described by the equations of calculus. And when it lands—BLAM!

Allegra, my daughter, who is also a neurologist, said I should measure the effectiveness of each breast implant research paper by the number of decapitated rabbits that arrive after each publication. We'll call that the Allegra Patten standard of scientific effectiveness. I was hoping by the time I was finished with the breast implant companies, I would have a whole hutch of dead rabbits and a closet full of crutches and duct tape.

* * *

Baylor College of Medicine Takes an Official Stand against the Limo

I loved the limo. It was a great productivity tool. Convenient too. In the limo, I could return the patients' calls and find out what was what with them. As a general rule, patients who get a callback come back. Patients who do not get a callback do not come back.

A Limousine Gets Attention

Trent and I liked the drama of arriving at the county hospital, Ben Taub, where I did my charity work four months each year.

As I exit the limo, a big black mama shouts, "Mister, you's at the wrong hospital."

"It's OK, I'm a drug dealer."

With that, a strange thing happens. Without anyone initiating it, the crowd stands aside, opening a long aisle to the front entrance. A young man with an AIDS face smiles and opens the door. He bows as I pass by and says, "Thanks for coming, Doc." He looks up and says it again, "Thanks for coming." Again, I feel like crying. This guy looks so sick and so pitiable. Yet, he is thanking me. The thought passes my mind: "Some researchers have to get working on an effective treatment for AIDS. Guys like this guy need a break."

The Limo Gets Me a Tax Deduction

Internal Revenue Service allowed full deduction of the cost of the limo from my income because I proved that the limo was my traveling office. They (there were two of them: a man and a woman for this, my 43rd income tax audit and my first field audit), also allowed full deduction for the Walther PPK 380 semiautomatic I carried: "Doc, we didn't realize medical research was so dangerous. No question, you need a gun. It's a business expense."

Some Baylor Faculty Disliked the Limo

The limo irritated people.

Bill Butler, president of the Baylor College of Medicine, called me into his office to tell me about it.

Bill: "Faculty members have complained about the limo. They think it doesn't look right for a doctor to arrive in a limo."

Me: "Why not? Alice arrives in a limo." (I was talking about Alice R. McPherson, the very famous Baylor College of Medicine retinal surgeon.)

Bill: "I won't go there. How about you have your driver let you off two blocks from the school, and you walk?"

Bill's idea of reasoning together was the equivalent of discussing the ownership of a side of beef with a Bengal tiger.

Me: "I … er … don't think that would be wise. I usually have patient charts in hand. The limo is my most important productivity tool. In it, I fill every unforgiving minute with 60 seconds worth of distance run. (Bill did not recognize the quote from Kipling.) Besides, it's normal for multimillionaires to travel by limo. I am doing the normal thing."

Entre nous, at the time it seemed stupid for the president of a medical school to waste his time, and my time, on such a trivial issue. But I was not then so well acquainted with his Lordship's character, of which stupidity was one of the strong features. Later, Snooty Bill sanctioned blocking my breast implant research (letter dated April 17, 20, and 22, 1995 available on request). This was a clear violation of the principle of academic freedom for tenured faculty members. It is hard for an empty sack to stand upright. Suppression of free inquiry is a cruel, dirty, and inexcusable anachronism.

For this sin, and many other problems, I believe Baylor College of Medicine deserves to lose its accreditation.

Baylor College of Medicine Placed on Probation

With satisfaction, I note that in 2013, Baylor College of Medicine was one of five medical schools in North America placed on probation for "14 areas of concern." Consult Professor Google for the details. The negative evaluation came from the Liaison Committee on Medical Education (LCME) formed in 1942 by the Association of American Medical Colleges and the American Medical Association. LCME evaluates 158 medical schools in the United States and Canada. The citations against Baylor College of Medicine included inadequate documentation of policies in regard to tenure, failure to provide safe environments for students from hazards, a need for better policies involving admission committee conflicts of interest, "every department" failure to timely report grades for students and supervise clinical rotations, a need for new processes to provide feedback to students, annual formal review of graduates, and a mechanism for faculty to contribute to decision making. More recently, Baylor and Saint Luke's Hospital are under investigation and have already received sanctions from the government about poor patient care, especially with transplant surgery.

Whew! All this and they are worried about some jerk arriving at work in a limo! My take on the situation is that the problems of Baylor College of Medicine are not correctable without divine intervention.

TV Adds to the Breast Battle Blues

"Bernie, It's Lennie. Sorry to wake you. Do you know CNN is camped outside your house?"

"Jesus fucking Christ! I told them no interview. They are trying to do an exposé on rich doctors exploiting the sick. Overcharging, over-treating—that sort of thing. So far, I cost the implant companies $4 billion, so they're after me."

"You bet. Bernie, there's four of them: cameras, crew, and trucks, and everything. Vince checked their credentials. CNN with press cards. One looks like he has AIDS, another is drunk, the other two seem angry. Should I call the cops? The mayor is your patient, and Vince is police commissioner. Say the word, and those guys are gone."

"Thanks, Lennie. I'll think about it. I don't want to cause a fuss. They'd probably film the cops. It might look worse for me if I had them removed. It might look like I was hiding something. You know TV. It's complete bullshit."

"Let me know if we can help."

I lay in bed, thinking about the options. I could sneak out the back, go down to the lake, cross behind the totem pole and into the neighbor's property. I could have Linda, my chauffeur, pick me up by the park. Or I can just go out and face them, tell them again no interviews. Or I could really give them a story. In fact, I could stage my own media event. After all, I have the Calico. Rather, I have two Calicos—each with a helical magazine containing 100 9mm shorts. I've wanted to test it on someone. I could come out shooting with both hands. In 20 seconds, spray every-one. That would make lots of dead meat. And something real for a change for them to show on TV. Or how about the Street Sweeper, I almost forgot about that, my au-tomatic shotgun, holds 12 12-gauge three-inch magnum shells. Hitting them with that would be fun and would, in fact, sweep them off the street. To them, the Street Sweeper would not only be an automatic shotgun; it would also be their gate to Hell.

I could see in my mind's eye, the lead reporter's chagrined face as he tries to stuff his guts back into that three-foot hole in his belly. Wow! I'd probably make the New York Times again, and the Wall Street Journal, and Time. But is that moment of fun worth the consequences? The food's not good in prison, I have heard. Also, I wasn't really sure I could get twice daily conjugal visits.

No violence unless provoked, I decided. I'll save the argument of lethal force as an item of last resort.

So, I dressed in my blue denims, my T-shirt with the Texas star, put on my stars and stripes socks and my flag cap with the red, white, and blue spangles making me look like the Vietnam-era veteran I am and decided to face CNN.

But before I went out the door, I slipped that gun blue Walther PPK 380 semiau-tomatic in my right front pocket. The police said I should carry it in view of all the death threats. And I've gotten used to feeling its heft against my leg. I find it reas-suring. Besides, it might help in my citizen's arrest of CNN for trespassing. People might not pay attention to me, but they will pay attention to the Walther, and when the Walther speaks, they'll listen.

As I approached the cameras, I waved, smiled a big cat smile, and shouted, "If you are watching, you are damaging your brain. TV is junk food for the mind!"

The next day, my patients in Malaysia and India called and said I looked great on TV! And my friend at Baylor asked why I mooned CNN. "I didn't moon them, Dave. I just bent over to pick up the Wall Street Journal, and my cheeks happened to point their way."

CNN voiced over what I said. Truth hurts, and the TV people knew what I said was the truth. They were not interested in truth. Instead, they were into hysteria, overreaction, and collective suspension of judgment. Eek! I was getting, by osmo-sis, a reasonable view of what was going on and what kind of real trouble would follow.

Doctor Patten Appears on Frontline

A program called Frontline was aired by WGBH in Boston. My friends told me it made me look very bad, like a perfect failure, and WGBH had voiced over what I said about TV being junk food for the mind with the following statement: "Doctor Patten is currently under investigation by the FBI for Medicare fraud."

That was news, especially since I had dropped out of Medicare long before. Medicare never paid enough, and they tended to be too picky about what they would pay for and what they would not pay for. The drop out was good for me. My income climbed the year I dropped out of Medicare. Why would anyone investigate a doctor for Medicare fraud when that doctor wasn't participating in the Medicare programs and wasn't billing Medicare for anything? Not possible! Conclusion: TV had lied.

FBI Does Not Investigate Medicare Fraud

One of my friends from a creative writing class at Rice University, a special agent of the FBI, said the FBI does not investigate Medicare cases. That is the job of the Office of the Inspector General (O.I.G.). She also checked with the agency and assured me that I was not under investigation by the FBI for anything, nor was I under investigation by the O.I.G. for anything. The record showed I had dropped out of Medicare and was not billing the government for anything.

Hot dog! Morris Hamm, my lawyer, my friend, and also a fellow student in the creative writing class at Rice University, and I were going to have a field day making money on this caper. The TV had told a lie about me to defame my character. For that lie, they must pay and pay plenty. I enclose a copy of Morris' letter to the TV station's attorney (letter). Here's part of what he mentions in his letter of March 19, 1998 to Eric Bass of the legal department of WGBH TV Boston:

Morris, My Lawyer, Writes a Nasty Letter

"It is clear to me, as it will be clear to a jury, that the program is not only maliciously unflattering to Dr. Patten but false in its accusations. The tone of the program, as evidenced early on, is that Dr. Patten prescribed expensive and unnecessary treatment for his patient, treatment that was to be paid by Medicare/Medicaid. Later in the program, the false allegation is made that Dr. Patten is under investigation for health care fraud and abuse by the Federal Bureau of Investigation as a voiceover onto old footage of entering a limousine. The fraud investigation allegation is used to buttress the prior allegation of unnecessary treatment. Further, it appears that the entire program is intended to malign the plaintiffs, their counsel, and their physicians for seeking recompense for the palpable injuries suffered as a result of the reckless behavior of certain companies in developing and marketing silicone breast implants."

"Dr. Patten's professional reputation has been impugned, and he has been maligned. He has suffered the loss of professional standing and suffered personal embarrassment and humiliation. The losses continue, as you have placed the program into the stream of commerce through replays and videotape sales."

"I am prepared to file suit on behalf of Dr. Patten against WGBH, the producers of Frontline, and all others involved in this libelous program. Prior to filing this suit, I am offering WGBH and the other potential defendants the opportunity to settle for a payment of $2,500,000, payable in exchange for a full release."

CNN Adds to the Breast Implant Blues

What WGBH did was bad but not as bad as what CNN had done. That program, aired in 1995, showed a woman who said I had treated her very badly. I had given her strong medicines that had caused multiple side effects and much pain and suffering. The Department of Neurology at Baylor was unable to locate that woman in any of the databases of the department, the medical school, or of the hospitals where I admit patients. I did not recognize her, even though she said I had given her all those expensive and dangerous medicines. Conclusion: she wasn't my patient at all. She was a fake. She was a shill.

But How Could We Prove They Knew She Was a Shill

The real question was whether the producers of the program realized she was just an actress pretending she had been my patient, or they just thought she was really a patient of mine who had just shown up out of the blue on their doorstep to complain about me. Also, in the same program, there appeared a man who claimed he was a rheumatologist. He didn't look like a doctor. He looked like a phony, and he sounded like a phony. He had trouble pronouncing medical terms, including the rheumatic disease systemic lupus erythematosus. The fake rheumatologist said he worked for Baylor College of Medicine and was a member of the rheumatology division of the Department of Medicine. He was unknown to that department and to the rheumatology division and was not registered as a physician in Harris County or Texas. Conclusion: he was a fake. He was a shill. How can TV get away with this kind of bullshit?

Answer: they can't.

They can't get away with it if they attack someone like myself who is willing and able to fight back. I have a feeling that the vast majority of people hurt by TV do not have the flexibility, the resources, or the time to fight back. I wasn't a myasthenic patient on a respirator or a stroke victim who couldn't talk. I wasn't an average schmuck muddling along in the survival mode, unable to fight back. I might look like a pussy, but I am not. I am an SOB (son-of-a-bitch) and was going to prove it. Following the example of my brave chauffer, Linda, I don't take no shit from nobody.

TV Settles with Doctor Patten

WGBH paid. The amount is sealed, and I am not allowed to tell you how much it was. Morris got his share and retired. The Bridge over Troubled Waters, in those days a charity safe house for abused women, got the entire amount that I received from WGBH as a gift from me to them to help abused women. The Bridge benefited from my charity, and I benefited from the tax deduction I got for the contribution. Morris told me WGBH offered sincere apologies, and they fired the producer of the program.

Other Media Encounters Add to the Breast Battle Blues

Talking about the media reminds me of other encounters I had with the media.

January 15, 1996, Michelle Nicholasen, associate producer, called me and asked me to help do a show about breast implants. I agreed on the condition that at the end of the program, they would give me two minutes and 30 seconds airtime to address women and tell them why I thought they should not get breast implants. I made this agreement with Michelle, even though I knew she was in the media business and wanted to sell her product. To make it sell, she had to make it interesting, and that meant controversial. In addition, from the way she talked, I knew she was going to put a negative spin on my work. But that wouldn't matter because during my time, I would look so sincere, so intelligent, and so knowledgeable that all the negativity would cancel, and most women would follow my advice.

American TV already broke down many boundaries between private and public information in its confessional talk shows so that they could exhibit human oddities and social outcasts and follow the examples set by the old circus sideshows. Not satisfied with that, they make up stories and stage events like those cars bursting into flame. So why should they not do a show about breast implants? And while at it, why not exaggerate and embellish the tale to keep those binge viewers interested and watching out there in TV land. Why let truth interfere with a good story? Reason and truth would take a back seat to emotion and melodrama. The information density would be slight, and some content would not be real. Oh well, reality is nice to visit, but most Americans can't live there and wouldn't want to live there even if they could. That's one of the reasons people watch TV—to get away from the realities of life. In modern America, we have escapism on a planetary scale.

Not All TV Added to the Breast Battle Blues

To be fair, CNN did two favorable programs about Britta Ostermeyer and me and our work, as did French 2, and German National TV. So, not all the TV coverage was bad or unfair. My patients in Malaysia and in Italy told me that I looked great on TV and that I am the most recognized American neurologist in their countries. All in all, if you measure things by the TV standard, we, Britta and I, came out ahead.

Michelle the Nasty's Interview Adds to the Breast Battle Blues

The third-degree encounter with Michelle, whom I now dub Michelle the Nasty, occurred in Honolulu.

Time wounds us humans with a fatal wound. And time wounded Honolulu, also fatally. Downtown looked like any other crowded American city. Here, the American dream had turned into a nightmare. The old Honolulu that I knew as a boy, where the airport had no building, just a tarpaulin to shield the tourists from the sun and rain, and from under which some nice young ladies dressed like real natives offered free leis—that Honolulu is gone forever.

The Hilton Hawaiian Village where Ethel and I stayed in 1971 now resembled a busy airport with people checking in bags and rushing about. It did not resemble the sacred haven of leisure that we once knew and loved. In the hotel's lobby, opposite the American Express travel desk and the local events desk (now selling luau tickets), I pushed through the crowd looking for Mike Day, the cameraman who was supposed to meet me. The tourists were supposed to be on vacation relaxing, but they looked frenetic. Why?

After the third hour of interview (interrogation would have been a better word), I asked Michelle the Nasty if it were time for my two minutes and 30 seconds. Yes, indeed! And I gave it my all and felt that I sounded good and sincere. Getting that message across was worth all the trouble. Now millions of women would think twice about getting breast implants. My speech was outstanding. My Uncle Bernie, formerly a New York State Senator, had trained me up to it.

Mike dropped me back at the Hilton, where I milled about making sure I wasn't followed. When the coast seemed clear, I took a limo back to the Queen Elizabeth 2. I was trying to make sure the TV people didn't know I was on Cunard's 1996 world cruise Voyage to Distant Empires, an experience subsequently published by Prometheus in my 557-page book, *Cruising on the Queen Elizabeth 2: Around the World in 91 days.*

Security Doesn't Stop Limos

Because we are a limo, they don't stop us at the gate where they stop regular taxis for inspection. Instead, they flag us right up to the gangway where I made a dramatic entrance with several passengers and crew looking on. Thank God the TV cameras are nowhere in sight. This is one time where I outsmarted them. Ho ho ho.

Wait a second! *What the deuce*! They are here, and they are filming me again as I get out of the limo. Once again, I shout, "If you are watching this, you are damaging your brain. TV is junk food for the mind."

TV Fools Me Again

The show aired and, as expected, Frontline made me look bad, as outlined in Morris' letter. Next time I make an agreement with TV people, I will make sure the agreement is in writing. It never occurred to me that they wouldn't air my 2 and a half minutes, but those lousy bastards didn't. My speech didn't fit in with the impression they were trying to make. They were comfortable deceiving the viewing public, so why should they not be comfortable deceiving me? What a fool I had been to trust them!

Cruising on the Queen Elizabeth 2 toward Sydney, Australia

Aboard ship, multiple faxes came—the usual and then one that was unusual. At 6 a.m., waking me from my habitual sleep of the dead, the radio officer from the bridge called. "Sorry to wake you, sir, but we have a fax here. We don't know who sent it, and we don't know where it is from, but it says, "You are bleeding!"

Blood is a Bad Word to Our British Friends

Queen Elizabeth 2 is a British ship. To Americans, "You are bleeding" doesn't sound like much. To the British, anything concerning blood, bloody, or bleeding is just about the worst swear word you can use. That is why the radio officer sounded so jangled by the message. I thanked him. I told him to expect more like that, and I asked him not to bother me with them. Then I rolled over and fell asleep. At home, we got anonymous calls, including death threats. At sea, we got anonymous faxes. All that must mean I am doing my job. I was doing my job, just as my father, Pop, did his. If Pop wasn't afraid of death threats from some criminal, I wouldn't be afraid of a bloody fax from some anonymous coward. See the letter I sent to Doctor Mark Donohoe, president of the Australian Comprehensive Medicine Association (ACMA), from at sea aboard the QE2.

The Australian Medical Society Gets Hit with the Breast Implant Blues

Doctor Mark Donohoe, the president of the ACMA, invited me to lecture when the Queen Elizabeth 2 arrived in Sydney. The lecture took place at the Darling Harbour Convention Center on Saturday morning, February 17, 1996. (See the official program among the accompanying documents.)

Donohoe said in his fax: "My organization is under mounting pressure." The Australian government had continued its support of a conference on the safety of breast implants, but the breast implant companies, including Dow, refused to participate. Dr. Donohoe said, "Your story and aloofness have done the predictable thing and created an almost insatiable media demand."

Donohoe was starting to get a feel for pressure. His office had been "invaded" with computer viruses, and confidential documents had been viewed. He was also dealing with a boycott from the plastic surgeons who were pressuring the Australian government regulator (Therapeutic Goods Administration or TGA, the Australian FDA) to drop its support for, and attendance at, the conference. And, oh great!, Dow's PR firm, Comber Consulting, and their apparatchiks had been faxing around "dirt files" and U.S. newspaper clippings on the U.S. speakers on the program. One file mentioned I was an "operator," meaning, I suppose, manipulative. In America, that is not exactly a compliment, but in Australia, it meant skillful and clever in a very good laudatory sense. I was delighted to learn this and continued to be amused by the slippery differences between Australian, British, and American idiomatic English. Some American newspapers said I was an operator and implied that was bad. The same clippings down under in Australia mean I'm good.

Donohoe said, "I have been roundly threatened with legal action by plastic surgeons, and a professor of medicine said he would sue for bringing 'these discredited charlatans and turkeys' from the United States. The adjectives used to describe you are astonishing. You are called impulsive, reckless, callous, and egotistical."

"Sounds like some people are irritated. I have been called worse. Nevertheless, as Willy Loman's widow observed, 'attention must be paid' even in a frosty and ill-spirited atmosphere—attention must be paid. I am used to dealing with hyper-moral editorial judgments and sanctimonious posturing based on mere conjecture and genuine ignorance. Sad to say, most of the critics haven't the slightest idea of how solid our medical research is or how long we have been working on implant problems. We can't walk on water, but we do know what's what. As surely as the sun sets in the west, we will be vindicated."

"You had better get yourself a good lawyer. Conservative medicine has closed ranks. Although I (Donohoe speaking) had invited over 3,000 doctors with an interest in the field of breast implants and their benefits and complications, only about 60 would attend the meeting. "

Disaster loomed. I could feel it in my bones. The medical association would be out many thousands of dollars if the attendance didn't pick up.

"On a somewhat better note," Donohoe said, "We have the full support of Senator Crowley, the Australian Minister of Health and in charge of the Therapeutic Goods Administration. And, believe it or not, Australia's premier comedienne and beauty myth smasher, Ms. Wendy Harmer, will launch the conference and introduce you and some of the other American speakers."

Donohoe had some advice for me: "Show yourself a flawed hero. That's what Australians go for. They don't mind charlatans as long as they are heroic."

"How about turkeys?" I asked. "Do they mind turkeys?"

"American slang. No one here knows what it means," he answered.

Flawed? No problem. I am flawed. Flawed hero? I don't know about the hero part. I shall just act natural and be myself. I have no choice. A round man can't fit into a square hole right away. He needs time to change his shape. Besides, I wanted to bug corporate America the way I bugged the brothers at Chaminade High School. For me, it was too late to change. Besides, there was something about insubordination and getting kicked out of high school that the Australians loved. Me too. I liked to shake things up. I liked to pull down the powerful. The research was done. The papers published. They had pissed off a lot people. That's that. Facts are facts. Those facts should be generally known. You agree?

Sometimes You Have to be Quixotic

"The moving finger writes and having writ moves on. Nor all thy piety nor wit can lure it back to cancel half a line, nor all thy tears wash out a word of it," says tent-maker Omar Khayyám. Our research papers are published. It is too late to change a single line or cancel half a line.

Tilting at windmills sometimes means that you are attacking powerful enemies or engaging in a hopeless cause. It's quixotic—the impractical pursuit of idealism. Until he was filled with pity for the galley slaves and for the whipped child, Don Quixote was alone, surrounded by strangeness, by the craziness of the world. In his *Meditations on Quixote* Ortega y Gasset wrote, as at the center of his reflections, "I am myself and my circumstances," which I understand as a symbiosis of two things. It is also a dilemma expressing those things as separate and distanced but interrelated. That's the reality. Cheers!

The lecture goes on after a stunning introduction by Ms. Wendy Harmer, who called me "a modern-day hero." Not a flawed hero, mind you, as I am, but just a modern-day hero. She may have been talking to some of America's plaintiff attorneys who think I am in fact a hero, their hero, their "6-billion-dollar" hero.

My lecture went well. The slides showed some breast implant disasters. No question about that. The real question is, how common are the complications? I couldn't say because I was seeing a select group of women who had implant problems. Britta's lecture went well also.

We left the podium under thunderous applause. Other papers that were presented showed the same or similar findings. That's what is so nice about research. It is like chemistry. You add silver nitrate to a sodium chloride solution, and you predictably get a precipitate. You put calcium carbide in water, and you predictably get acetylene. You add zinc to Drano, and you predictably make hydrogen. But sometimes you get an explosion that you had not planned. The explosion was what happened at the press conference right after my lecture. I hoped the reporters would ask intelligent questions and not engage in ad hominem. Wrong from the start!

The Press Conference Adds to the Breast Battle Blues

From the beginning, the press conference took on an adversarial tone. I tried to keep cool, but the questions focused on me personally and not on the research findings. This is a diversionary argument to focus attention away from the truth and onto irrelevant issues. The reporters preferred to concentrate on controversy rather than on the evolving set of scientific facts. They usually do have trouble distilling complex data. Telling the truth would require much more work than they were prepared to do. Negative critiques, disdain, and ignorance are easier, much easier, and have the added advantage of selling more papers. I was particularly downcast because I should have expected as much. Stupidly, I thought the press here in Australia would be different from that in the U.S.

Attack the Other Side's Experts

My father was a lawyer and taught me a lot about the law. In arguing a case, if the law is on your side, argue the law. If the facts are on your side, argue the facts. If neither the law nor the facts are on your side, attack the other side's experts. And that's what they were doing at the press conference. Britta and I were expert witnesses against the breast implant companies, and we were under attack, merciless attack.

Doctor Patten is a Socially Marginal Person

Question: "A neurologist at Mayo Clinic said that, as far as he is concerned, Dr. Patten is a socially marginal person who has always functioned on the fringe of society."

"Who is this guy who is knocking me down?" I asked.

The reporter looked puzzled. She is supposed to ask the questions. "We don't know. The statement was made anonymously."

"Oh! You don't know. Too bad," said I. "I was just curious to know if this guy had been talking to my wife. If you do find out who he is, let me know. I want to cross him off my Christmas card list."

No response. Instead, the reporter looked baffled. I was feeling better, more relaxed. This was good preparation for the writing career I had planned, learning how to handle hostile criticism and ad hominem arguments. The sky looked as though it might not fall any time soon. Chicken little is wrong.

Sad but true: as medicine became big business, as competition grows fiercer, it is common to hear doctors or hospitals knocking one another in an effort to get more money by recruiting more patients. Houston Methodist Hospital routinely, in a massive public relations and advertising campaign, claims they don't just practice medicine; they lead medicine.

Doctors need to be more charitable to one another. This unknown doctor from Mayo Clinic should not be bad-mouthing me or my colleagues simply because he/she does not agree with my research findings or my particular approach to breast implant complications. Besides, as a simple courtesy, they should at least give their names so I know who is talking and might be able to engage in a reasonable dialog about their complaints. Furthermore, how can I cross them off my Christmas list if I don't know who they are?

That anonymous Mayo Clinic person, I can tell, doesn't like me, and, truth be told, I don't like Mayo. Somewhere in this book to come, I will comment about the Mayo Clinic study of patients with implants, because it is a good of example of what I think is junk science.

Doctor Patten Used Dangerous and Expensive Treatments

Next question: "Isn't it true that *The New York Times* reported that you used expensive and dangerous treatments on sick women?"

Whenever a question starts with "Isn't it true" the answer that you should give is usually "No, it is not true." But I couldn't state that for sure because I didn't know whether it was true or not. I doubt the *Times* would print something like that. But the truth is I didn't know if they did or not. The question is also leading because if I said it was not true and they show the article, then they proved I am a liar. If I said it was true, then it would seem that I was admitting the conjecture and had used dangerous treatments.

In one of my reckless Irish moods, I answered: "Did you want me to let them die?"

The reporter, obviously irritated by my Irish way of answering a question with a question, decided to ask another question: "Why is the Baylor College of Medicine not affiliated with a university? Isn't that typical of inferior medical schools?"

"Whew! I thought we were supposed to talk about breast implants and the complications of breast implants. This is the first time I have heard that question, and it is a good one. My answer is I don't know. Baylor is loosely connected with Rice University, and I think negotiations are underway to tighten that connection."

Are You a Shit Scientist?

Question: "Isn't it true that the president of the European Plastic Society called you a 'shit scientist.'"

This is a complex question that would not be admitted in a court of law. If I said yes, people might not know what I was agreeing to—the shit part or the part about the president saying it or both. If I said no, then I would be stooping to their level and lying to make myself look good. In logic school, we call that a complex question and the way to answer it is to unpack and reply to the unpacked parts.

"It wasn't the president of the European Plastic Society that called me a shit scientist. It was the president of the American Society of Plastic Surgeons that called me a junk scientist. Junk and shit are two different things. Next time, try to get your quotes right.

"At the time, I think the president of the American Society of Plastic Surgeons was speaking in Europe. But, you know, in a sense, I am a shit scientist. That's what I have been studying this past decade—a piece of shit. That is what the breast implant was and is—a piece of shit!"

No Reporter Had Read a Single Scientific Paper

"By the way, did any of you read our published medical papers? Raise your hand if you have read a single paper that we have published in the scientific peer-reviewed medical literature."

No hands.

"Did any of you read the Department of Health and Human Services, Food and Drug Administration notice of the known complications of implants dated Thursday, September 26, 1991, a summary document that discusses capsular contracture, calcium deposits, rupture, silicone spread, changes in nipple and breast sensitivity, and interference with detection of cancer?"

No Hands

"Please take a look at the document. It has a nice discussion of the possible risks of autoimmune disease and rheumatic disease in patients who have implants. I have a copy in hand here. It is the Federal Register Vol. 56, No. 187, page 49,099."

No takers.

"Any of you want to see the Federal Register of January 8, 1993 on the same topics? It runs six pages of problems with the implants and has 51 references."

No takers.

"How many of you know Britta and I received awards for our clinical research from the Southern Medical Society and from the Texas Neurological Society. Raise your hands."

No hands.

But the big fat guy in the front row says, "No, and we have no interest in reading anything of yours. And we don't care about awards or the FDA. We've read the American newspapers and seen on TV everything about you we need to know. The Mayo Clinic Study is enough for us."

Ho ho ho. That's the man from Comber Consulting reciting his lines. I remember from other press conferences. Sad but true, there is a segment of the population that thinks if it is seen on TV, then it is OK and real. This time I'm ready. Let's see how Comber handles a curveball.

"Excuse me, Sir." (I impolitely point my index finger at him.) Have you read the Mayo paper?"

No voiced reply. He shakes his head—no.

"Has anyone here read the Mayo report? Raise your hand."

No hands.

"Does anyone here, besides myself, know the title of the report from Mayo?"

Again nothing.

"Does anyone here know what medical journal published the Mayo paper?"

No hands and lots of shrugged shoulders.

"Does anyone here, besides myself, know who paid for the Mayo study?"

Nobody.

"The Mayo paper, for your information, reports the result of chart reviews where the incidence of unspecified rheumatic disorders are counted in woman patients at the Mayo Clinic and compared to women patients at the Mayo Clinic who had implants. That study did not look for or count complications of breast implants. Thus, the Mayo study did not mention any of the numerous complications like the ones I just showed you in my lecture and the ones reported in the official notice from the American Food and Drug Administration.

What they should have done at Mayo is compare the number of local complications and redo operations in the implanted women to any other group of women, sick or well. Then, and only then, would they have found zero complications of breast implants in patients who did not have an implant, and they would have found about 30% complications, many serious, among the women who did have an implant.

"As journalists, you might consider doing some actual work to uncover the facts before you write up conclusions. And it may interest you to know where the money came from for the Mayo study."

I hold up the Federal Register. "Please read the American Food and Drug Administration's view of the implants as published Friday, January 8, 1993, pages 3,426 to 3,443. FDA says the implants cause all of the local side effects I mentioned in my lecture, and they add the side effect of infection and deflation. The FDA says the manufacturers failed to test silicone for safety and failed to inform women of the dangers of the breast implants. The FDA also says it believes the silicone may cause autoimmune and rheumatic diseases. The FDA gives in the Federal Register Part X, 51 references about complications of breast implants from the medical literature. Most of the references are from the Journal of Plastic and Reconstructive Surgery."

Ugh! I was getting ugly and being smart, and even worse, I was repeating myself. I really need to calm down. Time to throw in the towel. This group is hopeless. They don't know anything, and they don't know they don't know anything. And they don't want to learn.

If they had been nicer, I would have told them about the deflation problem, which is also described in the Federal Register. I had such a patient. She called on the weekend, telling me she had to have her deflated implant replaced.

"Can't it wait until next week?"

"No, my husband is out of town, and I was with my lover, so I need to get fixed up before my husband gets back."

"Which breast?"

"The right."

"That's unusual. Usually, it's the left implant that ruptures because the man is squeezing with his right hand."

"My lover is lefthanded."

I took a long last look at the Australian press boys and shook my head. Never give an Irishman an excuse for vengeance. I decided to tell them off.

"You people are just wind, no real substance. And your moral sense is wonky. VERY WONKY! If you don't know what the word wonky means, look it up.

"None of you are interested in reasonable dialogue. You are hacks. Hack writing is, simply, writing for money, just as contract killing is killing for money, and prostitution is sex for money. You know you are a hack writer if you say in print what you don't believe or what you haven't checked."

"I will brook no more questions. I have better things to do. Good day."

They would edit my answer. But that would not change the good feeling I have about the conference, Doctor Donohoe, the Australian Medical Societies, Senator Crowley, Ms. Wendy Harmer, the Therapeutic Goods Administration, and Australia.

Back on the QE2

Nathan, my old professor, who taught me how to read cardiograms, spotted me. "You are all over the news tonight." Nathan patted me on the right shoulder. "Australian TV was very favorable to you." Then he told me why. "Australians love a flawed hero, you know, especially those who show lack of respect for authority."

Alex Seymour, the manager of Queens Grill, came over to our table. "Are you the very famous Doctor Patten the news is talking about tonight? They even filmed someone who could be your twin brother swimming in the ship's indoor pool."

"Not me, Alex, but while you are here, please tell Simon (Simon was my private bartender) to bring me a Black Bush on the rocks. Make it a double."

Ethel kicked me under the table. She said, "Since when have you become so modest?"

"I want to enjoy dinner, and I don't want them lining up for autographs."

Max Bygraves tried to cheer me up with a few stories:

"A nine-year-old went into a chemist's shop and said, "Three condoms, please, Miss."

"Don't you miss me."

"Right. Make that four condoms."

"A woman asked her physicians about breast implants. "Don't get implants," the doctor said. "They might have consequences." (Consequences is the British for side effects.) So, the doctor gave her a magic mirror, which she addressed at home. 'Mirror, mirror on the floor... make my breast size a 44.' Bong! It happened. She showed her husband. While she was away to get a larger bra, her husband tried it. 'Mirror, mirror, on the wall... make my ding-a-ling hit the floor.' Whereupon, the tires fell off his bicycle."

"Come on, Max, how about it? Try to tell a funny joke," says I.

"A Catholic priest went to London and walked along the West End. Some ladies of the night came up to him and said, "Try a quickie, Gov'nor for five quid." Further down the lane, another lady came up and said, "Five quid for a quickie." The priest refused again, but he realized he didn't know what he was refusing, So when he got back to Dublin he called the Mother Superior in the convent next door and asked, "Sister, what's a quickie?" "Five quid same as London."

Sidebar about Mayo Clinic

In 1994, we heard much of the music of a study from the Mayo Clinic published in the New England Journal of Medicine entitled "Risk of Connective Diseases and Other Disorders after Breast Implantation." The implant manufacturers claimed the study confirmed with scientific certainty that the silicone implants do not cause connective-tissue disease or, in fact, any disease. The paper is available. Those of you who are interested should read it and come to your own conclusions. Here I state my objections.

Objection One

The control group consisted of 1,498 women who were patients at Mayo Clinic. Their health was compared by chart review to 749 women with breast implants. 10

women in the control group were identified as having a connective tissue disease and five in the implant group. A much better control group would have been normal women matched for age, not women who were sick enough to go to Mayo and were already enrolled at Mayo for treatment. Why did Mayo select sick women as the control group to compare their health to that of implanted women? It doesn't make sense. A better control group would have been normal women. That way, if there were a difference in health between the normal women and implanted women, we might make some reasonable conclusions about whether or not the implant caused disease.

Objection Two

None of the patients who had implants were actually examined or tested for the purposes of the study. We don't know how many of them had implants for cosmetic reasons versus how many had implants following breast cancer surgery. The follow up of patients consisted of assuming the patients were well if they did not appear again at Mayo. No attempt was made to contact these patients by mail, or phone, or questionnaire, and no attempt was made to obtain subsequent medical records to see if the women were well. It was assumed they were well when they could have moved or had gone to some other place for treatment. Some Mayo refugees did come to Houston for treatment, and some of those patients were very sick. Those former Mayo patients would have been counted as healthy because they didn't go to Mayo again.

Yes! From the date of last visit at Mayo, a woman with an implant was treated as "healthy" and not needing or receiving any further medical care. The authors would not even know if the patient had died if she had not died at Mayo. Conclusion: follow up of the patients was poor. Due to the poor follow up, any conclusions about the health or non-health in the implanted patients are moot.

Objection Three

The study was negative. Negative evidence is not conclusive of anything. If you see it, you can believe it. If you don't see it, you don't know. It could have been there, and you missed it. Absence of evidence is not evidence of absence. If I say I see no bacteria on my pillow, and I am looking with a telescope and report "no bacteria." I have used the wrong method for finding bacteria. I should have used a microscope and reported billions of bacteria. If the Mayo study had looked at local complications of breast implants, they would have found, like most researchers, migrations of the implants, ruptured implants, infections, capsule formation, calcifications, inflammation, rare lymphoid tumors (like anaplastic lymphosarcoma—over 400 cases and 16 deaths so far in the U.S. from this unique cancer that starts at the edge of the implant), and multiple redo operations. Over a 10-year period, you can expect local complications in at least 30% of breast implant patients.

If I close my eyes, I can see magnified images of those big, clumped, massive collections of lymphocytes at the edge of the removed implants. God knows I made superbly detailed photographs of the collections. The fact that some lymphocytes could turn malignant was a problem I might well have sorted out while still doing the research. It escaped me, and I must now bow to progress.

Objection Four

At the meeting of plastic surgeons in New Orleans, I presented my data and the interesting case of a woman who received a blood transfusion into her breast implant. The intravenous catheter in this patient had been misplaced into the implant and not into the neck vein where it was supposed to be. The patient complained, as the first unit of packed red cells was running in, that her breast was enlarging. The nurse assured her, "that is impossible." During the second bag of red cells, the implant ruptured and spilled silicone and blood into her chest tissues. This situation was similar to the patient report by Varga in Annals of Internal Medicine, 111:377-383, 1989 in a paper entitled Systemic Sclerosis after Augmentation Mammoplasty with Silicone Implants.

In the breast area of the spill, my patient developed a dense fibrotic process, which some pathologists called scleroderma or systemic sclerosis, and some pathologists called dense fibrosis. The fibrosis spread from the breast area, encircled the chest, and traveled concentrically from the breast to involve most of the body leading to respiratory insufficiency and death.

At the same plastic surgery session, the Mayo physician presented her data, which included a group of patients in the implant group who had autoimmune thyroiditis. After the session, I talked with the Mayo epidemiologist, who told me that I was right. They had confirmed an increase in autoimmunity in the implanted patients and an increase in rheumatic symptoms, including muscle stiffness, morning stiffness, and joint aches. The increase in rheumatic symptoms did appear in the final paper, but the thyroiditis cases were not mentioned. Why? The high incidence of rheumatic symptoms was in the Mayo paper but not discussed in their paper or in the news articles about the paper. Why?

Furthermore, I was told Mayo researchers initially reviewed 971 medical records of women with implants. They excluded 149 because they did not meet criteria, but my friend, the epidemiologist, did not know what criteria they did not meet. Then the Mayo researchers advised PSEF (Plastic Surgery Educational Foundation of the American Society of Plastic and Reconstructive Surgeons) that there were 822 women left in the study, but the published paper refers to only 749 women. What happened to the 73 (822 – 749) implanted women who met criteria but who do not appear in the paper? Did they have diseases? Why were they not included in the paper? We may never know.

Objection Five

Despite the severe limitations of the Mayo study, Dow Corning ran full-page advertisements in the New York Times and the Wall Street Journal about the Mayo report. On October 13, 1995, on the Oprah Winfrey Show, the CEO of Dow repeated the claims implants were as "harmless as water," citing the Mayo study as evidence. This behavior was irritating because the companies seemed to be taking their public relation moves from the tobacco company playbook, trying to convince the public their product was harmless when they knew it wasn't. Company executives knew or should have known that, sooner or later, the truth would come out, and there would be a day of reckoning.

The connective tissue issue (whether implants cause connective tissue disease) was a diversionary argument, a red herring, to focus attention away from the facts about the local complications of implants. I had never said implants caused autoimmune disease or connective tissue disease. The companies were constructing a straw man to blow over. Although it has not been scientifically proven, I believe some patients will react to silicone such that the silicone becomes an adjuvant that promotes the development of autoimmunity. Britta and I had taken care of hundreds of patients who had both autoimmune disease and breast implants. But we couldn't say for sure that the two items (autoimmunity and implant) were related as cause and effect, although it did seem they were. More research is needed to know for sure.

Meanwhile, Britta and I were confident about what we had seen. We had hundreds of patients with terrible problems with their implants, we had hundreds of positive laboratory tests showing disease states, and we had hundreds of pictures of ugly, deformed, inflamed breasts, and we had many pictures of gigantic spills of silicone goo during the explant operations. Ours was not conjecture or mere assertion. We had the facts, and we were right. Fact trumps all arguments to the contrary.

Objection Six

The Mayo paper says the study was funded in part by the Plastic Surgery Educational Foundation (PSEF). In fact, that is true but misleading. Dow and the other manufacturers gave PSEF the money. PSEF funneled the Dow money to Mayo. R. Barrett Noone, MD, chair of PSEF, stated in the multidistrict litigation, September 7 and 9, 1994, that PSEF was the "facilitator" to deliver the manufacturer's money to Mayo. That information is part of the transcript and also part of a written communication to me from attorney Stephen A. Sheller who did the deposition. Mayo should have disclosed the real source of their funding, but they never did. If it had been generally known that Mayo got implant company money for its report, some people may have found the study less believable. It would be interesting to know who exercised final editorial control of the Mayo paper, and it would be interesting to know who actually reviewed all the charts. It is hard for me to believe the charts were actually reviewed by physicians. That would have taken lots of time and energy. Most chart review papers are the work of interns, residents, or fellows and not attending physicians.

As for our research, Britta and I turned down a $50,000 grant from plaintiff attorneys of Houston because we felt it would have posed a conflict of interest, implying we might not have been entirely objective in our analysis of our data. The truth is that our research was supported by Mr. George Lindler, a Houston builder who was in remission of myasthenia gravis due to our treatments. Mr. Lindler had no vested interest in breast implants. He was just a nice guy who wanted to do some good with his money and wanted to see his name in print on scientific papers.

Objection Seven

Mayo was a defendant in the lawsuits brought by women who had received their implants at Mayo. That fact was not mentioned in the published paper. I think the Mayo paper should have mentioned the lawsuits. If the implanted patients were doing so well, why were they suing? And what were they suing about? We will never know.

Back to Australia
Australian Newspapers Hammer Me

When the papers came out the following day, the storyline that had been prefigured by Dow and Comber Consulting was featured. There was no way to change it. Truth and fiction, as we understand the distinction, don't sometimes exist in the media. It is all narrative, narrative, narrative—augmented by the usual journalistic failing of assigning too much importance to the things reported and, of course, narrative shaped by bias. And the bias is shaped by (what else?) money, often very big money from corporate treasuries. Oh well, what do you expect? Some journalists (the minority) are and will probably always be professional slingers of hyperbole and bullshit. If I sound down on Australian journalists, it is because I am. They were mean to me, and I am returning the meanness.

Gina Kolata had done the same thing in the United States, in my opinion. She, as an excellent science writer for the New York Times, should, in my opinion, have known better and looked deeper into the situation. She was intent on writing a great story—one that would sell newspapers, one that her editors liked. She and her editors may have actually believed they uncovered the truth about breast implants, while Britta and I, who had been studying the complications for over a decade, had been fooled.

But, how much of her story and the story written by other reporters had to do with my impatience with the press and their questions? The answer is probably unknowable, but I see reporters as more interested in "capturing the controversy" than in learning the truth. They had no consistent set of objections, only a never-ending stream of quibbles, no matter how convincing our data or how startling our clinical pictures of breast implants gone wrong.

The Old Tricks Work

What gets me is that the public believes the merchants of doubt like Comber Consulting. The old tricks really work! We are seeing the same thing in climate change denial. There is an unholy alliance of corporations, partisan politics, pseudoscience, and marketing that has given climate change denial some traction, despite cogent scientific evidence and consensus. History teaches lessons. I recall the days when lead in gasoline, according to the people who put it there, was OK. DDT manufacturers and tobacco companies pushed back critics by falsely claiming their products did no harm. With the help of Hill & Knowlton, public relations, the false tobacco claims were passed as fact. Eventually, truth won out. The companies had to pay billions in settlement for the diseases they caused and the lies they told.

Advertising Pays

All the ads and spin about breast implants paid off. The general public, after massive PR, thought breast implants are just fine and dandy, and the women who have them should be happy and not gripe or complain. Will truth about breast implants win out? What's your bet? How will this story end?

Before we get to how it ended, let's take a look at how it began.

Nostalgia Ain't What It Used to Be—How the Breast Research Got Started

One fatal day, I decided to leave the sacred groves of the National Institutes of Health to take a job as chief of neuromuscular diseases, and eventually vice chairman of Neurology at the Baylor College of Medicine in Houston, Texas.

Doctors Gerow and Cronin

At Baylor, I made friends with Dr. Frank Gerow, one of the two inventors of the silicone breast implant. Frank explained that he and Dr. Thomas D. Cronin wanted to do something with plastic surgery that would match the artificial heart that Dr. Michael DeBakey was working on, something that would draw national attention to themselves the way NASA, situated only 40 miles south of Baylor, got national attention.

First, they tried direct injections of silicone into tissues to make bigger breasts, and the results were, of course, a disaster. I saw these women in consultation. They were, by and large, the wives of medical students who had volunteered for the experiments. The silicone caused marked fibrosis, hard, painful, disgusting looking breasts, which the women were ashamed to show. All others who tried to inject silicone into human tissue have gotten the same terrible local complications, proving that silicone is not inert, but is biologically active enough to cause severe local inflammatory reactions.

> **Lesson:** Direct injection into any human tissue is a no-no.

The direct injection of silicone into human tissue causes a special type of gangrene known as "silicone rot." The direct injection of silicone into any human at any time for any reason is now illegal throughout the United States of America and in most countries of the world.

The Women I Saw with Silicone in Their Breasts Were Sick

The interesting thing that escaped my attention at the time was that most of these wives also had weird neuromuscular and rheumatologic diseases, including myasthenia gravis, polymyositis, small fiber sensory neuropathy, and Sjogren's syndrome. In many cases, the autoimmune diseases required treatment, and I applied the treatments the best I could without thinking that there might be a connection between the silicone and the autoimmunity. I had not yet had a glimpse of the reality or of my destiny. I was too stupid to connect the dots and too focused on the individual patients and their problems. I missed the forest for the trees.

The Silicone-Filled Bag is Invented

Because direct injection gave awful results, Doctors Gerow and Cronin decided to enclose the silicone in an elastomer bag and put the bag into the breast area to make big breasts. A lot of people thought the idea absurd, almost obscene, but it did give the promise of what some woman wanted, and it was quick, giving immediate results. Of course, there were lots of problems with the surgery, including infections and herniation of the implant through the incisions and multiple redo operations because the implant had ruptured or shifted or had developed a baseball-hard capsule, or the women wanted still larger and larger breasts and so forth. But the local complications Gerow and Cronin could handle. Besides, whether you put implants in, or took them out, or changed them, the surgeon still got paid.

Baylor College of Medicine Becomes the Mecca for Those Seeking Fake Breasts

Eventually, Baylor accumulated the first and the largest series of implanted women in the world, and, as the neurologist that Gerow knew and presumably trusted, I got the referrals of the women who had complaints referable to muscles, nerves, spinal cord, or brain. And there were many of them, a superabundance. From 1986 to 1993, I personally saw and examined many such women. Their stories were all similar: sometime after the implantation, they felt weak and tired, developed morning stiffness, excessive fatigue, dry mouth, dry eyes, and dry vagina. Most also had hot, painful, tender breasts with contractures. I made it my business to examine the breasts of all these women and got pretty good at detecting ruptures, spills, and enlarged local lymph nodes.

Anesthetic Nipples Surface as a Complication of Breast Implants

There were many women with anesthetic nipples. They felt nothing when their husbands or boyfriends touched or licked or sucked their nipples. Why?

Gerow told me the nipples were anesthetic because T4 (the fourth thoracic nerve), the nerve to the nipple, had been cut on insertion of the larger implants through the axillary approach. Quite a few of these women had severe sharp shooting chest pains simulating heart attacks when their breasts were squeezed. Gerow had an answer for that too: on insertion the implant forms a physical barrier to the regrowth of severed nerves, causing neuroma formation. We even biopsied the chest area in a few cases and proved that neuromas were present and published two papers on chest pain in implanted women. One paper appeared in *Emergency Medicine*, and one appeared in *The Southern Medical Journal*. But the thing that impressed me the most about the local situation was that the implant, in this selected group of women that I saw, had failed miserably to deliver what it had promised. Beautiful breasts, they were not. In fact, the opposite was true. The implant had made satisfactory breasts horribly deformed and ugly. But, of course, I was seeing only the women where things had gone wrong. There was a group out there that had good results and liked their bigger breasts. This was especially true among women who were showgirls, exotic dancers, and prostitutes.

Silicone Breasts are a Big Plus for Exotic Dancers

The exotic dancers told me their bigger breasts increased the size of their tips tenfold. Big tits = big tips. One exotic dancer was actually saved by her implant. An 86-year-old man had fallen in love with her. When she rejected him, he shot her in the chest with a .25 caliber Beretta. The bullet bounced off the implant, which had a very thick elastomer shell, in fact, the thickest in the business: the Jenner. The Jenner had an elastomer shell so thick it was bulletproof. The Jenner also had the additional advantage that the thick shell prevented the small molecular weight dimethylsiloxane from leaking into tissue. This small molecule caused local inflammation and probably is the cause of the stimulation of the immune system in some implanted patients. Future implants would probably do well to have thicker shells and thicker gels to prevent leaks and to decrease the local and systemic side effects. But, then, of course, the implants would feel even more like rocks than they do now.

The Companies Attack

The companies, through their attorneys, claimed the implants did not leak silicone. That was silly. I never had a problem proving the Dow implant leaked silicone. I would simply take the new implant fresh out of the manufacturer's box, place the implant on a flat surface, wait two minutes, then pick it up. Always and without fail, the implant left a film of silicone on the tabletop. As you can imagine, plaintiff lawyers had a field day demonstrating the leaking implant to the juries at trial.

I did complete physical examinations on each of the sick women referred to me and found they all seemed to show much the same general pattern: they had skin rashes, cold fingers and toes, dry eyes and dry mouths, and they were weak. We weren't sure how strong a woman should be, so I sent out a medical student to get pinchometer and gripometer measurements in normal and hospitalized women. The results confirmed that implanted women, the ones referred to me, at any rate, in relation to their peers matched for age and sex, were objectively weak, usually scoring less than 50% of the controls on the dynamometer measurements. On neurological examination, I found the ladies had more than the usual trouble with simple mental status tests, such as proverbs, subtractions, serial sevens, naming the presidents, and so forth. That could have been because they came from poor education backgrounds, which they did, by and large. Except, even some high-powered women who had completed graduate school, judges in Houston courts, for instance, or the former assistant postmaster general of the United States and other women of achievement in journalism and science, also did poorly on these tests. Gait and station testing showed most couldn't do a push-up or a sit-up, and most had glove and stocking sensory loss, suggesting they had neuropathy. All this did not add up to any known disease but did seem to be a syndrome associated with the implants. If you were looking for some kind of typical autoimmune disease in these patients, you wouldn't find it. Multiple epidemiological studies have proven that.

Laboratory Results Indicate Autoimmunity

Laboratory tests confirmed the women had something autoimmune, though just what that was we couldn't say. There were lots of abnormal auto-directed antibodies including ANA (antinuclear antibody) and rheumatoid factors and anti-nerve antibodies, but none of the ladies actually fit into the currently accepted diagnostic criteria for the diseases usually associated with those antibodies. Almost all the women who had cognitive complaints had decreased cerebral blood flows, as measured by research physicians, as part of the NIH-approved Baylor-Methodist Cerebral Vascular Research Center grant. Almost all had positive tear tests, proving objectively the ladies really did have dry eyes.

Explant the Implant

Most of the patients had surgical indications for implant removal—rupture, spill, encapsulation, migration, herniation, and so forth. I followed the patients during and after the surgery. I reviewed the slides on all tissues removed and gradually learned to identify free silicone in tissue, polyurethane, and the dense inflammation with foreign body giant cells that surrounds the implant. I was concerned about the massive collections of lymphocytes around the edge of the implants. If just one of those lymphocytes turned nasty, the patient would have a malignancy called lymphoma. Now (2019), we know the implants can and do cause cancer. FDA has 414 cases, and 16 women have died of implant-associated anaplastic large-cell lymphoma. So far, the cancer developed exclusively in women with textured implants, but FDA thinks it could develop in relation to any implant. FDA also thinks the number of reported cases (414 and 16 deaths) is an underestimate due to poor reporting. Me too. I think it is merely the tip of the iceberg, and I predict the longer the implant stays in a woman, the more the lymphocytes accumulate, and the greater the chance of malignant change.

Britta and I documented, with pictures, the gross appearance of massive silicomas and capsules thicker than magazines. We kept track of the relation of examination results from before to what happened after surgery. In general, women with polyurethane implants did lousily and got worse after explanation. Women who had massive spills of silicone had teams of surgeons laboring over nine hours fail to get all the silicone out. That group also did poorly. Women with high titers of antiGM1 antibodies got progressively worse, and some died of a weird neuromuscular disease that resembled a combination of dermatomyositis, lupus, rheumatoid arthritis, motor sensory neuropathy, Sjogren's syndrome, and amyotrophic lateral sclerosis with, believe it or not, signs and symptoms of multiple sclerosis! Women who had minor spills that surgeons could remove and those with intact implants did the best. Most in that group recovered within two years. We don't know what the lab tests did in this group because we did not repeat the test. If the patient is normal, why do a test? Three of these recovered women who had had complete remissions of well-documented diseases got tired of living with small tits and made the mistake of getting reimplanted. The diseases roared back. That made a believer of me.

Example: one 17-year-old girl with severe myasthenia gravis went into remission with the appropriate treatments. Two years later, despite my advice, the woman now had implants. The myasthenia roared back. Removing the implants restored the remission and the patient is now 61 and still in remission from the myasthenia, but she does have metastatic cancer of the breast.

We found that the incidence of ruptured implant correlated with the severity of autoimmune disease. The proven rupture rate for our series of severely ill women with the multiple-sclerosis-like syndrome, for instance, exceeded 70%, and most of those patients had antiphospholipid antibodies in their blood. We published our results in eight papers covering everything we could think of, from the local to systemic problems. The citations of all papers appear in Medline and were all peer-reviewed. My fellows, Britta and Glen, and I presented our data at national and international meetings, including the World Federation of Neurology, the American Neurological Association, and the American Academy of Neurology.

The Southern Medical Society and the Texas Neurological Society, as mentioned, gave us awards for clinical research and encouraged us to dig further. In many cases, our reports hit the front pages of *USA Today, The New York Times, The Wall Street Journal*, and so forth. Little did I realize the publicity would hurt us. Nor did I realize, until it was too late, how much it would hurt, and how much real trouble and suffering from company-sponsored vengeance was headed our way.

The Implants Had a High Rupture Rate and Too Many Complications

Dow-Corning paid me to consult with them about their product. I told them what we were finding, and I told them especially about my concern about the rupture rate (50% ruptures in 10 years on average) and the severe local complications we had seen due to ruptures. At the time, I was concerned about the leaking silicone, but not that much. I urged them to apologize and set up some form of free clinic to care for the injured women and to make cowardly amends for what they had done. Some months later, they told me I was wrong and that the implant caused no such problems. After all, Frank Gerow had told them that the implants were "as safe as water."

Breast Implants Were Not as Safe as Water

In view of what Dow told us, we went back to the drawing boards and redid much of the research, only to discover the same things we had discovered before. I estimate the pause caused by the misinformation received from the company delayed our progress for two years. And it was misinformation because, to my chagrin, I learned on my way to Washington to testify before the expert panel of the FDA, while reviewing the secret company documents supplied to me by FDA, that the company clearly knew as far back as 1975 that silicone leaked out of the implant, traveled through tissues, caused local inflammation, and, as far back as 1976, they knew silicone implants resulted in autoimmune diseases and death in experimental animals, especially dogs.

Tableau Thirty-Two:

Breast Implant Adventure— the End

Company Documents Show a Cover-up

The company documents had been subpoenaed by the FDA. And WOW! They sure made the companies look bad. When an experiment went wrong, that is contrary to what they wanted, the scientist signed a confidentiality agreement and often added a note to say why the experiment came out wrong. "The implants were placed in non-breast areas in these dogs; therefore, the migration of silicone and the development of autoimmunity can't be taken as relating to humans." Statements like that were funny and sad. Ignoring evidence is an error in logic because it tends to focus attention away from the truth and toward error.

The Federal Drug Administration (FDA) Supplies 8,000 Pages of Documents

My two fellows, Mavis and Glenn, tried to wade through the more than 8,000 pages supplied to us by FDA, but never got through them all. Mavis picked out pages she thought I ought to read on the plane headed to Washington, D.C. It was all there, of course, the leaking silicone, the migration of the implants, the encapsulations, and the activation of the immune system. In addition, there was a conference in which some executives suggested hiring two hit men from San Diego to kill me and make it look like a suicide. I assume this was said in jest. But who knows? It isn't every day that you see in writing that someone wants you killed.

FDA Conference

I appeared before the panel a shaken man. The people who had hired me as a consultant had deceived me. How naïve I had been. Of course, the first thing I said to the FDA panel and to the hundreds of reporters and all those TV cameras was:

"I am not about to commit suicide."

That statement seemed weirdly out of place at a scientific conference. But in light of what I read in the company documents, it was important to me to get that idea out in the open. I was trying to avoid the fate suffered by my environmental officer from Beaumont and suffered by Silkwood from Oklahoma.

"Before I start, I want to make one thing perfectly clear: I am not about to commit suicide. If I am found dead, assume I didn't kill myself, and please find out and bring to justice those who did kill me."

Dow Has a United States Patent That Silicone Stimulates the Immune System

After the FDA conference, a man in an elevator handed me a paper. "Here," he said. "This will interest you." He was dressed in gray, wore a fedora, and looked like he was out of one of those grade-B spy movies from the 1940s.

The paper was a copy of a patent awarded to Dow for the use of the low-molecular-weight silicone as an adjuvant to vaccines. The patent claims that the silicone increases the antibody response to the vaccine, and the paper had data to prove it. Thus, not only did the company know that their product stimulated the immune system, they had patented the effect for future use and profit. The company was caught in a contradiction because they were officially claiming their low-molecular-weight siloxane did and did not stimulate the immune system. They said silicone did stimulate the immune system in the case of vaccines, and they said it did not stimulate the immune system in the case of their leaking breast implants. How's that for a contradiction?

The other problem was the warning in the package insert that came with the breast implants. The company said that if an autoimmune disease is present or suspected, then the implant should be removed with the surrounding capsule, and such patients should not be reimplanted. Further, the package insert said implants should not be placed in patients who have autoimmune diseases. If the companies felt their implants did not cause or worsen autoimmunity, then why did they put those recommendations in their package insert?

I saw myself on TV at Washington National Airport. Some people look better on TV than they look in real life. And some people look much, much better on TV than they look in real life. That's me. On TV I looked great!

The Rest, as They Say, is History

FDA, concluding the device was not safe or effective, took silicone implants for cosmetic augmentation off the market for 14 years. The general immunological and pathological principle is that any foreign material placed into the human body will be detected by the immune system, and a rejection reaction will occur. How severe and what kind of rejection will depend on the substance placed and the individual genetic makeup of the recipient and the duration of exposure. Not every woman gets the autoimmune complication, and I venture to say most women do not. But those that do suffer.

Spin, Misinformation, and Counterattack

The implant companies reacted harshly. They spent millions of dollars on public relations and spin, creating the illusion in the public mind that the implants were OK, but, of course, they never explained why the FDA said their product was not safe or effective, and they never explained why the FDA took their product off the market.

Texas Medical Board Gets a Host of Anonymous Complaints

Multiple investigations were conducted on the basis of anonymous complaints to the Texas Board of Medical Examiners. All seemed to claim that Britta and I were endangering the public health. Some of the complaints seemed reasonable. After all, we were dealing with a new form of illness and a previously not fully recognized complication of the breast implants. We were trying to find our way, and we were using new ideas that people had a right to question. But most of it was blue smoke designed to tie me up and waste my time and energy. The claimants wanted the board to censor me or limit my license or perhaps take my license away. The chance of that happening was slim. Some of the anonymous complaints were insulting. I bore the insults as best I could and fought back, representing myself and not hiring a lawyer. Britta and I kept exact and detailed records of every patient. The records discussed in extenso the reasons for the treatments and so forth. The records proved we were reasonable scientific doctors.

When the board asked Stanley Appel, the Neurology chair at Baylor College of Medicine, what he thought about Doctor Patten's practice. Stan said, "His practice is on the edge, but within the standard of care." The board thought that meant I was on the edge, the frontier of medical science, and doing a great job as a researcher, but I wonder if that is what Stan meant.

Texas Medical Board Dismisses All Complaints

On April 12, 1999, the board dismissed the latest (number nine) and last complaint against me. That last claim was about the medical care of three patients I knew loved me, so the complaint could not have come from them. Indeed, I learned during the hearing of the case the complaint came from a person in the employ of and paid by the implant company, Dow. None of those patients even knew about the complaint. Dow had complained to the board without the knowledge or consent of the patients! What despicable little odious vermin.

Company Lawyers Attack

It wasn't fun enduring all those investigations, but the Texas Board was a kitten compared to attorneys working for the breast implant companies: every 35mm slide I ever showed in any scientific meeting was seized by implant company attorneys and investigated as possible evidence against me. They found nothing: no made up data, no fake patients, no misread slides. Britta was meticulous in her research, and the lawyers for the implant companies proved how careful we had been.

Baylor College of Medicine Joins the Attacks

Baylor restricted my teaching, saying that they couldn't prevent my research, but they sure could stop me from talking to students, interns, and residents about implants. They were careful to mention that they were not restricting my teaching in any other area or my research because they recognized the rights of a tenured associate professor to publish what he wished. And they affirmed that they wished me to continue my Baylor job in every other aspect, just as before. However, the chairman of the department, Stanley Appel, soon came upon the idea that he could stop my seeing implanted women. I protested this indirect way of stopping my research, but Baylor administration remained intransigent, saying the whole area was too controversial, and Baylor itself was being hurt by all the suits against it.

So, realizing the futility of trying to make further progress, I bowed out. Here, we had a medical college that was supposed to be dedicated to patient care and research stop, for economic and political reasons, the care of a particular type of sick patient and the research thereon. My resignation letter contained a handwritten note by Baylor's president, Doctor William Butler. Read the letter and his note and draw your own conclusions (see documents attached).

Note: I never believed the rumor that Baylor got $3,000,000 to stop my research, though many people did believe it.

Thomas Cronin Dies

Meanwhile, the nurses told me that Cronin started to make rounds in the nude and was discovered to be demented. Thomas died October 21, 1993, at age 87. He was a fine surgeon and had pioneered major advances in the surgery of cleft lip and palate.

Frank Gerow Dies

Frank Gerow, drinking a lot, refused to have his Protime checked. He had an artificial aortic valve for which he took Coumadin. He claimed that he could tell when the Coumadin dose was too much by how long the paper cuts bled! He was a fine surgeon and had made major contributions to plastic and reconstructive surgery. His subsequent death prompted me to formulate the following epigram:

The silicone implant was:

Bad for those who made them

Bad for those who put them in

Bad for those who got them in

And bad for those who did research on them.

God rest his soul. Before he died, Frank Gerow predicted what subsequently came true: "The silicone implant, born in Houston, will die in Houston."

All Malpractice Cases against Plastic Surgeons and Physicians are Dismissed

The malpractice cases against Gerow and Baylor were dismissed. Including plastic surgeons in the suits against the companies was a legal ploy to keep the cases in the state courts and out of federal court. Plaintiff lawyers thought they would do better in state court than in federal court and merely asked at the beginning of the cases that the defendants, Gerow and Baylor, and all the other doctors involved be dismissed.

Conclusion

Well, what finally happened? The media that had done such a good job of showing how bad our research was did a relatively poor job of informing the public of the final result. The FDA decisions against the companies were never fully covered, and the public was not informed about why the implants were taken off the market. The Wall Street Journal, to its credit. did explain the settlement and the facts about the cover-ups (see below).

Implant Companies Lose and Lose Big

Their product and their malfeasance cost them $6.2 billion. Plaintiff attorneys dubbed me the "Six-Billion-Dollar Man."

On September 2, 1994, *The Wall Street Journal* published the news of the final settlement approved by U.S. District Judge Sam C. Pointer, Jr. in Birmingham, Alabama. Judge Pointer said the global agreement was generally "reasonable, fair, and adequate." He cleared the way for women to file claims against the settlement fund. Nearly all major suppliers, manufacturers, and distributors of breast implants are party to the agreement. The leading corporate participants are Dow Corning Corporation, a joint venture of Dow Chemical and Corning, Inc., Bristol-Myers Squibb, Baxter International, Minnesota Mining & Manufacturing, and Union Carbide.

Women were to be, and are being, compensated for ruptured implants, spilled silicone, and a host of autoimmune diseases. You can read about the compensation plans on the internet by dialing the subject into Professor Google.

Implant Companies Found Liable on the Basis of Their Own Research

The Wall Street Journal article went on to explain that much of the evidence came from company documents (147 pages reviewed by Thomas Burton, Staff Reporter of *The Wall Street Journal*) that showed that as far back as 1975, the company knew about the immune effects of low-molecular-weight silicones. Much of the original work had been done on dogs at Dow Corning. When the experiments came out the wrong way, i.e., showing complications, scientists signed a secrecy agreement. And a lot of experiments in dogs did turn out the wrong way: that is, the experiments showed the silicone-induced autoimmunity. Furthermore, the company, as mentioned, applied for and received a U.S. patent for the use of silicone to augment the antibody responses of vaccines. Thus, Dow was caught in a contradiction. On the one hand, as I stated, they argued that the silicone had no effect on the immune system and yet, on the other hand, they argued in their patent that it did. Logically, you can't have it both ways. Either the dimethylsiloxane stimulated the immune system, or it didn't.

The Package Insert Contradicts the Companies

The other contradiction noted by the court was the package insert itself. The package insert came with the implants. The insert said, as I pointed out, that if a woman had an autoimmune disease or if an autoimmune disease was suspected, then that woman should not be implanted. If a woman develops an autoimmune disease after implantation, then the implant should be removed along with the surrounding capsule, and such patient should not be reimplanted.

Thus, the manufacturer is caught again. The court noted that if they didn't think the implant influenced autoimmune disease, why include in the package insert the advice that it could? Logically, you can't have it both ways. Either you believe your implant can influence the immune system, or you don't believe it can. If you believe it can, then you put that statement in your package insert as a warning.

In court, it looked like they knew in certain women the implant could cause autoimmune disease, and they had put a warning in the package insert to notify physicians of that fact. My own take is that is the truth. The company was trying to help physicians make reasonable decisions about who should not get an implant. Furthermore, the package insert even told the doctors what to do in the event that an implanted woman developed an autoimmune disease: explant the implant and the surrounding capsule (to remove the leaked silicone) and do not implant that woman again. By recommending the implant be removed and the capsule too, the companies showed they knew silicone leaked into the capsule of connective tissue that surrounds the implant.

Lesson: The thing that bothered me the most about the breast implant research was the reception the research received among my neurological colleagues. I was completely unprepared for their resistance. Many of them, including some in high places in the American Academy of Neurology, told me they were sure I was wrong. "Which of my eight papers do you disagree with?" I would ask. Not a single one of them had read any papers on the subject. They had gotten their information from TV! Thus, some neurologists were no better than other people who watch the boob tube. They, too, were gullible and misinformed! Their closed minds created a rather long and harrowing journey for me and Britta Ostermeyer lasting over a decade.

Court Cases are Complex

The court cases were interesting. Some women were obviously sick and harmed by the implants, and others were pretending they were harmed in order to get some money. Some women were harmed but exaggerated their suffering to get more than they were entitled to. Others who were significantly harmed and their families devastated never sued at all.

I found myself testifying on both sides of the fence, depending on the circumstances.

Breast Implant Companies Were Probably Like Other Large Organizations in America

Breast implant companies were an easy target for plaintiff lawyers. They kept good records and had both liquid and real property assets. The incidence of malfeasance was probably no more than that of any other comparable institutions in America. The sexual abuse scandal in the Catholic Church was a great tragedy and a largely self-inflicted wound. But Philip Jenkins points out in his study, *Pedophiles and Priests*, the actual incidence of sexual abuse in the Catholic Church and its school system is no higher than in other institutions. In fact, it is less than what exists in the New York City school system. This is not offered in any way as a defense. That such abuse should have existed at all is unforgivable. But this prompts the next question: why was the Catholic Church scandal the one that got so much attention from the media, public officials, and lawyers. Answer: the Church, like the implant companies, kept good records and had liquid and real property assets. They were an easy target and did not enjoy the special legal protections of the New York City School System. Plaintiff attorneys are well aware of this and, being practical litigators, took aim at the easy targets.

The real offense, of both the church and the implant companies, was the cover-up. Once the problems with implants surfaced, the companies should have addressed them directly and not tried to cover up. Once the priest problem surfaced, prelates should have addressed the problem directly and not tried to cover up. It is for the cover-up that penance is required and is being paid. Unfortunately, some of the people paying are completely innocent. My friend Leonard is a name of Lloyd's of London who helped insure the implants. Leonard has paid quite a lot because of implant defects, and he has suffered accordingly. The poor who would have benefited from the good works of the Church from the funds now depleted because of the misconduct of some churchmen have also suffered.

Baylor College of Medicine, the Department of Neurology, and the chairman Stanley Appel were wrong to silence me and the research on implants. For that sin against the Holy Ghost, they shall not be forgiven.

Testimonies

Hollywood stars have had problems with breast implants and have not been afraid to tell the public. Testimonies are selective and subjective and therefore, unscientific, but they do tell of interesting personal experiences and outlooks. Consult the reference below in the National Enquirer for details. The quotes are from that article by Patricia Towle, Don Gentile, and Marc Cetner.

Breast Implant Adventure—the End

Pamela Anderson Lee

According to Dr. Richard Ellenbogen, a Beverly Hills plastic surgeon, "Pamela Anderson had huge implants, and huge implants have a much higher complication rate. Pam felt uncomfortable with her large breasts and had them replaced by smaller implants. At surgery, one of the large implants was found ruptured with silicone spilled into tissue. When the large implants were removed, her breasts became saggy, deflated breasts, requiring uplift procedures and replacement implants. Thus, Pam went from 36DD to 36C."

Mary Tyler Moore

Mary experienced months of pain when her implants hardened following a 1991 procedure. Dr. Ellenbogen said, "In 95% of cases where women have their implants removed, it's due to the hardness phenomenon. The body reacts to the implant, causing scar tissue to form around it. To a woman, this feels like a knife in the chest." Mary was forced to undergo a second operation to replace the implants with new ones. She said, "If I'd known this was going to happen to me, I'd never have had the implants in the first place."

Jenny Jones

Jenny wanted a fuller figure—and instead wound up with "11 years of hell." Silicone implants the talk show hostess got in 1981 hardened, and five operations later, they still weren't right. So, in 1992, she had the implants removed. Her experience, which left her with breasts that are numb and asymmetrical, convinced her to start a foundation that urges women with implant problems to seek medical help. She said, "I don't have cleavage, but I am better off without them." Jenny went from 36C to AA. Jenny is famous for holding up her implant on her show while explaining that she thought they caused those "11 years of hell."

Cher

Cher survived several procedures. "My breast operations were a nightmare. They were really botched in every way."

Stevie Nicks

Stevie says she's "living proof" that breast implants are not safe. In 1994, the Fleetwood Mac songbird became weak. She suspected the implants she got in 1976 and had them taken out. "It turned out they were totally broken," said Stevie. She kept the removed implants in her freezer "to remind me of the agony."

Neurology Rounds with the Maverick

Sally Kirkland

Sally, the star of EDtv, had to endure nine corrective surgeries following the rupture of her silicone implants in the late 1980s. "My body became a battle zone of scar tissue from all the operations. And I was fighting the toxic die-off as the silicone moved through my body, poisoning healthy tissue. Sally's replacement saline implants fared no better, and they were removed in August 1998.

Mary McDonough

The child star on "The Waltons" developed lupus after receiving breast implants in 1984. She finally had them removed in 1994. She said, "not only had they ruptured, but the polyurethane foam around them had melted and seeped into my system. So, everything had to be scraped out."

Enough

That's enough sad stories about implants gone awry. In writing about these problems, I suddenly realized that the patients I talked about here with implant problems were women. Implants caused similar problems with men. One patient, the president of a South American country, had trouble with his butt implants. Another New York City cop had trouble with his muscle implants. A well-known TV personality seemed to develop an autoimmune disease and a local reaction to his cheek implants. Another man had problems with his testicular implants and so forth. My point is that men were also affected and that implant problems are not exclusive to women.

Suggestions

And so, it is with a kind of wispy regret that I make some suggestions to future scientists who might consider doing implant research on the new implants that are supposed to be safer because they have thicker shells and are made according to stricter standards. First of all, consider carefully, you men and women of the future, and if you take my advice, don't do it. It isn't worth it. Do not do any research that has anything to do with a device or medical product made by corporate America. More than one career has been ruined in this field, and others are sure to follow. The companies have massive amounts of money to defame even the most sincere and diligent researcher. The chance that you will escape the same fate as mine is slim. But if the compulsion to do research that will have a significant impact on health for our time and for all time is unavoidable, I suggest you consider the following:

1. Set up special free clinics to study the women and men with implants. These people have genuine medical problems which are not being addressed. Regardless of the cause of their physical and mental diseases, they need help, which they are not able to get at present because, for various reasons, they are locked out of the medical system.

2. Repeat the epidemiological studies. Most of those studies, by their own admission, are flawed.

3. Even forgetting about possible causation for the moment, why not study intensively the mechanisms of autoimmunity in patients with implants? At the time of my retirement, I had collected 51 cases of ruptured implants in patients with multifocal brain infarctions associated with antiphospholipid antibodies. Could that be an accident?

4. Follow all men and women with implants in a national registry. Require that all have yearly screening examinations for local and systemic complications. History and physical examinations are all that is needed for effective screening. Career researchers not connected with the companies in any way and not connected with the business of installing or removing implants in any way should do the screening. The companies have spent millions of dollars on spin to make themselves look good. Why not spend a similar amount on some real unbiased research? As a precondition to the licensing of the new implants, the companies promised to follow up on each implanted person to record the true incidence of complications, if any. That follow-up promise has not been kept, and the FDA seems incapable of making the companies keep it. The reporting of implant-associated, large-cell anaplastic lymphoma, a serious and sometimes fatal complication of breast implants, is voluntary. So, many cases of this malignant tumor are not in the registry. This explains why we know so little about this malignancy, who gets it, what implants are at fault, and what treatments work best and so forth.

References

B. Patten and B. Ostermeyer, Disquisition on Human Adjuvant Disease, *Perspectives in Biology and Medicine*, 1995, 38, 274-290.

Britta Ostermeyer Shoaib, Bernard M. Patten, Dick S. Calkins, Adjuvant Breast Disease: An Evaluation of 100 Symptomatic Woman with Breast Implants or Silicone Fluid Injections, Keio J Med 43 (2): 79-87,1994. This article has multiple pictures of implants ruptured. The pictures are not for the faint-hearted.

L. Lu, B. Ostermeyer, B. Patten, Atypical Chest Pain Syndrome in Patients with Breast Implants, *Southern Medical Journal*, 1994, 87, 978-984.

Plastic Surgery Breast Disasters: 20 Stars tell their story, National Enquirer, May 4, 1999, pages 28,29,32,33.

Farewell

Under happier circumstances, I would have liked to write a conclusion to this series of disconnected records. But I can't. The reason is that nothing has, in fact, been concluded. Wait a second. That nothing has been concluded is itself a conclusion. But you know what I'm driving at. In fiction, everything can be decided, including outcomes. Whereas here, in nonfiction, in the core chaos of real life, I can decide nothing, as I am entirely at the mercy of realities I can't fully encompass. And you, you dear reader, so are you.

We, the living, are part of an unfinished work in progress, unfixed, mysterious, and only half-conscious of our own ends. We will probably continue that way until it is too late.

So, why did I write this book? What was my purpose? What's the point?

My aim was to show you a world you didn't know. Did you see it? There are two main themes: 1. how things were in the golden age of medicine and 2. the important role of choices.

About theme one: this may have been a golden age for doctors, but for some patients, it was a gilded age, and for others, an ice age. More modern approaches to imaging the nervous system and the major advances in treatment speak for themselves. In my era, doctors had practically nothing to help cancer victims. That situation changed and is changing.

About theme two: choices you make set in motion forces in your life and in the lives of others. The future is not fixed. The future is contingent. By selecting some paths and rejecting others, you make the future. How would you have decided about not telling parents that their daughter smoked dope in the schoolyard? Would you have gone ahead with the removal of Ruth's spleen, despite the lack of informed consent? Would you have burned the diary of the old lady who needed hugs in clinic? Would you have had the guts to stand up to implant companies? How would you have handled the whistleblower who got murdered for his trouble? Would you have continued the normal pressure hydrocephalus evaluation and treatment of patient Callas, despite the fact that H. Houston Merritt, probably the foremost neurologist of the time, had advised the patient to sign out of the hospital because "the boys have bad things planned for you."

In my day, there were doctors who were not controlled by insurance companies, corporate medicine, or the government. In my day, medicine often, but not always, existed in a sweet, unspoiled atmosphere, ruled by a sense of service, wonder, and adventure. It was a medicine against the implacable and the unmerciful; it was a medicine that tried to overcome evil with good. And think about this: if in our world there is no transcendence, then we human beings have only each other.

But in my day, medicine was often ineffective. If I were still practicing medicine, I would wish medicine to be the way it was—kind, considerate, and personal. But as a patient, I'll take the more modern and more effective treatments and forebear the often-impersonal encounters. Perhaps in the future, we can have a compassionate medicine along with an amazingly effective medicine. That's my hope. The two modes are not mutually exclusive.

In my view, there is a real need to lower expectations in medicine. All those ads from Houston Methodist Hospital seem to say Methodist is the place to go because they don't practice medicine. They lead it. In this age of hype, that stuff has to backfire because patients will come to expect the impossible and will be disappointed. Houston Methodist must spend millions of dollars on ads, dollars that might have been better spent on charity care or medical research. Although I have seen many ads from Houston Methodist in the Wall Street Journal and in the Journal Neurology, never have I seen any of those ads picture a patient. The ads are about doctors looking at x-rays, or glaring into microscopes, or working in the laboratory. Scientific medicine is there. Humanistic medicine is not.

Another problem is the medical focus has shifted from attending the sick to protecting the bottom line by recruiting patients and bragging how good your institution compared to others. The objective of the system is cost containment to increase profits. An army of managers has been put in place to accomplish the profit purpose such that managers, lawyers, accountants, reviewers, etc. now outnumber the doctors. Result: the health care system is on a collision course with professional doctoring. Sooner or later, doctors will rebel. They will have to.

The other problem with the modern medical scene is hype about not-so-important problems. Cholesterol is the latest fad. Many of the tap dancers in my tap troop are healthy, robust women who are taking anti-cholesterol drugs. One woman showed me her lab report and asked my advice. Her cholesterol level is 202. The upper limit of normal for the laboratory is 200. Hence, her physician put her on a cholesterol-lowering agent. The first drug he tried caused too many side effects. Ditto the second drug. A month later, after drug three, the laboratory reported the cholesterol is 210. Now her physician wants to add another agent because he thinks the cholesterol has risen. There is no difference between a 202 and a 210. Those values are within the known error of the test. The joke is my tap dance friend is 77 years old and in great shape. Furthermore, the fractionation of her cholesterol shows her high-density cholesterol is nicely elevated at 76. Therefore, the reason for the 202 elevated value in total cholesterol is her high-density cholesterol, the good cholesterol that mobilizes fat from tissue, is high. To add insult to injury, because of the reported 210 cholesterol, her physician wanted to put her on a low-fat and low-cholesterol diet. This would be especially counterproductive, as it usually is in the elderly whose diets are already impaired by dentures, constipation, lack of appetite, and intolerance for many nutritious foods. I told her to ignore the advice, eat what she wishes, and forget about cholesterol. "You survived to 77. Your cholesterol won't make a hill of difference. Eat whatever you like. Besides, your cholesterol is not a problem. In fact, it is quite good."

Sorry! As you can see, besides showing a different world, on occasion, I got on my soapbox. Where my own judgment is given, the fact is clearly signposted. Cards of invitation. That's what the lessons in shout type were about. Go with what works for you, which may be different from what works for others or for me. Don't go with what doesn't work for you. You won't hurt my feelings either way. Focus on what matters, and forget the small stuff. And if you are like me, you will realize most of it is small stuff.

So that's that, dear reader. We met from different universes, overlapped. I came out having gained a certain experience. You did too. And experience counts. Despite my many shortcomings, my doctoring has improved some, and so has my judgment. Now I am more helpful to others than I was before.

If offered the choice, I should have no objection to repeating my life from its beginning, only asking the advantage authors have in a second edition of correcting the faults of the first. Besides correcting the faults, it would also help if I could have avoided some sinister accidents, pitfalls, and bad decisions and produced a more favorable outcome from my career as an academic physician. But all that is water under the bridge. I neither boast nor complain. I was younger in those days, fascinated with my work, and recognized its importance. It's too late for regret or resentment. Time and fate have changed me and the world. I shall never be young again. (But that fact doesn't prevent me from being my immature self as usual.)

And time, the real enemy of mankind, runs on. Already, I have lived most of my life. It's been a good run and an interesting experience, a happy time mainly. I am grateful to have loved human beings, including the imperfect and even sinful ones. I am prepared to face my fate. How about you?

Goodbye, and good luck!
Your friend,
Bernie

www.ingramcontent.com/pod-product-compliance
Lightning Source LLC
Chambersburg PA
CBHW071319210326
41597CB00015B/1278